Organic Fast Food Recipes

Kenneth C. Kozeka, Ph.D.
Julia A. Kozeka

To Julia A. Kozeka, whose love, inspiration, and meal
preparation made this book possible.

To Max Gerson, MD, Charlotte Gerson,
Caldwell B. Esselstyn, Jr., MD, T. Colin Campbell, PhD,
John McDougall, MD and Neil Barnard, MD
for their knowledge, courage, and humanity.

Contents

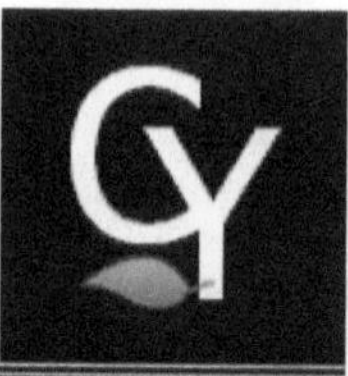

Preface

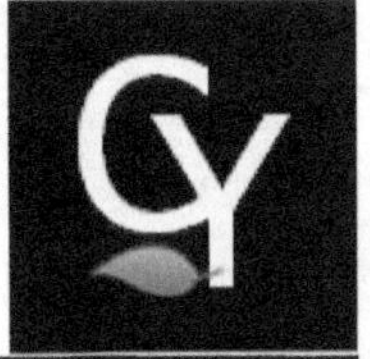

Over the past century, the U.S. and other industrialized nations have moved away from a plant-based diet to an animal-based diet that includes a lot of animal products and processed food. It has taken several decades for us to realize that the "standard American diet" is responsible for the horrific epidemic of chronic diseases that now causes suffering and early deaths in the U.S. and other countries. Despite my medical school education and chronic migraines, I remained oblivious to the effects of the toxic and nutrient poor American diet for most of my life. It was not until my wife's cancers returned many years after having the tumors removed that I gave serious attention to the relationship between nutrition and disease.

To help my wife restore her good health and avoid more surgery, chemotherapy, radiation treatment, and early death, I read many books and scientific papers and watched countless documentaries on nutrition and disease. My biomedical education and research experience made it easy for me to open my eyes and see the obvious, that proper nutrition is essential for proper cell function, a healthy immune system, and overall good health. I learned that less than 2% of diseases are due to genes we are born with and are instead caused by our diet and environmental toxins. I soon discovered that tumors are the symptom of cancer, not the cause of cancer. Removing the tumors does not remove the cancer. The tumors usually return as they had for my wife. It became apparent to me that the cholesterol in animal products clogged blood vessels causing heart attacks and strokes. To my surprise, I learned from Dr. T. Colin Campbell and other independent scientists that animal protein causes cancer cells to grow rapidly while plant protein does not. I was astonished by the fact that processed foods such as a slice of cake could contain as many as 60 ingredients, some that I could not pronounce and most of which are toxic to the body. I was appalled to discover that non-organic fruits and vegetables could each contain as many as sixty toxic substances that were known to cause cancer, disrupt hormones, damage neurons, and interfere with development and reproduction. It was now clear to me that an organic, whole, plant-based diet was essential for good health and to prevent the many chronic diseases that plagued the U.S. and other countries. Cultures that consume a plant-based diet rarely have cancer, cardiovascular disease, and all the other chronic diseases known to involve autoimmunity and the immune system.

It was a challenge to determine which vegan diet would provide the nutrients needed for optimal health to reverse my wife's cancer and her recently acquired weight-gain. I was drowning in an ocean of nutritional remedies and diets that usually involved recipes with a dozen or more ingredients. I found there are more than 300 diet and exercise books published each year and sold on Amazon. After comparing many diet plans, evaluating the nutritional content of foods, and applying the most widely accepted nutritional information, I concluded that a healthy diet is comprised of mostly complex carbohydrates and approximately 10-15% each of protein, fat and micronutrients (vitamins, minerals, antioxidants and phytochemicals). Eating salads for breakfast, lunch and dinner is not necessary to obtain an adequate amount of micronutrients, the most important part of a healthy diet. Carbohydrates, the largest part of a healthy diet, can be obtained from rice, potatoes, legumes and beans as advocated by Dr. McDougall. The carbohydrates serve as "fuel" nutrients used to produce energy for the body. Only a smaller part of the total diet must be organic vegetables or "super foods" such as kale and spinach that are loaded with the essential micronutrients.

With this acquired knowledge and the help of my wife, we were able to develop an organic, plant-based diet that is nutritional and affordable and with recipes that are quick and easy to make. I call these meals and recipes "Organic Fast-Food". An organic, plant-based diet does not have to be expensive, the recipes do not have to have 12 or more ingredients, and they do not have to take 1-3 hours to prepare.

Since we adopted an organic, plant-based diet, we have both been free of cancer and all other chronic diseases. Our body and mind now crave healthy food and reject animal products and most processed foods.

I am appalled by those who claim that switching overnight from the highly addictive standard American diet to a whole, plant-based diet is easy. It is not easy; for most of us, it is rather difficult. Switching your diet takes time and cannot be done successfully in a week or month; instead, it may take a year or more! If you try to make the switch quickly, you likely will not sustain the change, and instead, you will go back to your poor diet. It took several years for my wife and me to make a complete switch.

I decided to write this book to share the years of hard work that led my wife and me to adopt a healthy, plant-based diet that is tasty, affordable and easy to prepare, and that reversed all our diseases. This "organic fast-food" recipe book provides you with many simple, quick and inexpensive recipes. It is designed to allow time for your brain and taste to stop craving the bad food and start enjoying the good food. Your brain and taste buds will change in a few months to a year greatly reducing, if not eliminating your taste and desire for meat and other animal products, fast food and processed food. The delicious beef, chicken, sausage, and hotdog substitutes will help you overcome your addiction to animal products. The substitutes recommended in this book taste and look very much like the real meat and dairy products. I have conducted several "blind" tests and often the consumer did not realize they were eating a meat substitute. Some of the meals in this book, especially the ones with meat substitutes, are intended to help you move away from most or all real animal products. They are meant to work like methadone works for heroine addiction. The meat and dairy substitutes serve as a transition and do not represent the best vegan meals.

After you change your diet, you can eat nearly as much as you want without gaining an excessive amount of weight. No more calorie counting and feeling hungry all the time. There are no special foods or supplements, you only need to eat more organic, fresh plants. I hope you like this book and that it helps you switch to a healthier diet, bringing you good health and reversal of chronic diseases you may have. Over the past decade, I have helped many people change their diet and cure themselves of cancer, depression, asthma, arthritis, gallbladder disease, high blood pressure, cardiovascular disease and diabetes. If you make a significant improvement in your diet, you will enjoy a much happier and healthier life.

Please understand that organic plant food does not cure diseases. Organic plant food provides your body and immune system with the nutrients needed to restore normal and healthy function of cells, tissues and organs. If you are suffering from one or more serious diseases, the odds are good that if you switch to a 100% whole, plant-based, organic diet, all of your diseases will stop progressing, if not reverse, as it has for tens-of-thousands of other people for decades.

Introduction

Making it Easier to Switch to a Plant-Based Diet

The purpose of this book is to help you make a successful transition to a healthier, plant-based diet. Success means that you make a meaningful and permanent improvement in your diet and as a result, your health improves considerably. It is highly likely, especially if you switch to a 100%, organic plant-based diet, that the chronic diseases you may have will reverse, or at least stop progressing.

If you are in a terminal stage of cancer, cardiovascular or other disease, you must give up animal products and most, if not all processed foods, and adopt a 100%, organic, plant-based diet immediately. Thousands of people have reversed their chronic diseases, even when the disease was in an advanced stage, by switching to a 100%, organic, plant-based diet. Their plant-based diets varied considerably; some included lots of juicing and liver cleansing while others did not. The organic, fast-food recipes in this book alone are not optimal for reversing chronic diseases that are in a serious or terminal stage. They are intended to make your initial transition to a plant-based diet easier. If you are seriously ill, I strongly recommend that you make the green juice a major part of your diet, drinking six or more glasses each day.

Flooding your body with nutrients from juices is the most effective plant-based diet therapy and should be a major part of your new diet until your disease has subsided. If you are terminally ill, you should obtain guidance and medical support at a Gerson Clinic or from a practitioner trained by the Gerson Institute who can come to your home (www.gerson.org). The Gerson Institute also provides on their website a home program that you can do yourself. Other effective plant-based diet therapies are provided in books written by Dr. Esselstyn, Dr. Barnard and Dr. McDougall.

If your health is not in serious decline, you may not have to give up animal products entirely, although that would be best. Furthermore, every meal does not have to be a salad. Most of what we eat is used to produce energy. That energy should come from glucose, a carbohydrate. Glucose is intended to be the body's primary fuel. An organic, plant-based diet comprised largely of complex carbohydrates will provide the fuel nutrients your body needs. Potatoes, pasta, rice, beans and other legumes are a good source of carbohydrates for fuel and provide ample protein and fat. Fresh, and preferably raw, organic vegetables and fruits can be a smaller portion of your diet and will provide all the micronutrients (except vitamin B12) you need for good health, especially when made into a juice.

The first and most important task for you is to begin consuming all the micronutrients you need for good health. This can be done easily by juicing organic plants. It is the quickest, easiest and least expensive way to consume essential micronutrients. You must first put good nutrients into your body to restore proper cell function. Juicing is easy and should begin immediately. The first two recipes in this book are for juices that are easy to make and easy to drink. They will provide you with the micronutrients you need for healing and good health. If you are suffering from a chronic disease that has progressed to the point that it poses a threat to your life, it is important that you flood your body with plant micronutrients by drinking six or more plant juices throughout the day until the disease subsides.

The organic fast-food recipes in this book will help you move away from the standard American diet that is animal-based and includes lots of processed foods toward a healthier, organic plant-based diet with minimally processed foods. Fast food restaurants such as McDonald's and processed foods from the grocery store are convenient. Most of us have little time to spend preparing meals at home. With that in mind, most of the meals in this book can be prepared in under 20 minutes and some in under 10 minutes, about the same time it takes to order a fast-food meal. Most vegan recipes available on the Internet and in recipe books have ten or more ingredients, some of which are difficult to find in a store. The recipes in this book have 5 or less ingredients that are available in most grocery stores.

It is especially difficult for some people to give up meat and dairy products. Many of the recipes in this book include excellent tasting meat and dairy substitutes that taste, look and feel like the real meat or dairy product. These substitutes can make it much easier for you to reduce or exclude meat and dairy from your diet.

In addition to being quick and easy to prepare, the meals in this book are inexpensive. Most people believe that an organic, vegan diet is expensive. Yes, in general, organic food is more expensive. However, when you switch your diet, you will likely eat much less because the food you eat has a higher nutritional content which satisfies your hunger with less food. All the meals in this book cost $5 or less (per person), similar to the price for a meal from a fast food restaurant.

I strongly recommend that you use a toaster oven instead of a regular oven. A toaster oven is faster, cheaper to operate, easier to clean, and quicker to preheat. Most toaster ovens are large enough to bake bread, pies and a medium-size pizza. No need to heat up a large oven just to bake a couple of potatoes.

Typical American meals are huge. In time, the size and number of meals you eat each day will likely get smaller. Nutritious meals are far more satisfying and filling than nutrient-poor junk food. Many vegans, including my wife and myself, typically eat only one meal each day and have healthy snacks in the morning and evening. It is healthier to eat several small meals throughout the day than one or two large meals. A healthy "snack" can often be a full meal. Also, consider having for lunch or dinner some of the meals that you normally have for breakfast (and *vice versa*). For example, you could have pancakes and meatless sausage for dinner and a sweet potato for breakfast.

There are many excellent vegan recipe books and vegan recipes on the Internet. For example, Dr. T. Collin Campbell's Center for Nutrition Studies on the Internet (www.nutritionstudies.org/recipes) provides many highly nutritious vegan recipes with little or no processed ingredients. These and other vegan recipes typically have 10 or more ingredients including some that are difficult to find at the grocery store. Preparation time is often an hour or more.

This recipe book contains meals that are inexpensive, quick and easy to make and have few ingredients. Some of the meals are pre-cooked and frozen, and other meals include canned and minimally processed organic ingredients. Any micro-nutrients that might be missing in these fast-food recipes are provided for in the juices that should be a routine part of your diet. Consider this recipe book to be a bridge that helps you move away from the standard American diet toward an organic, plant-based diet. It is quite a challenge to abandon the standard American diet that is convenient and tasty and adopt a plant-based diet that requires giving up the foods you like and a lifestyle change.

Change is hard for most of us. Some find it difficult to switch to a plant-based diet even when we know it is vital to our health and well-being. The program in this book worked for my wife and me, and for many others. We hope it works for you.

Vital Juice Recipes

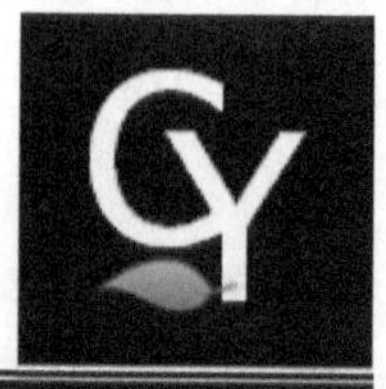

Providing Vitamins, Minerals,
and Antioxidants That You Need

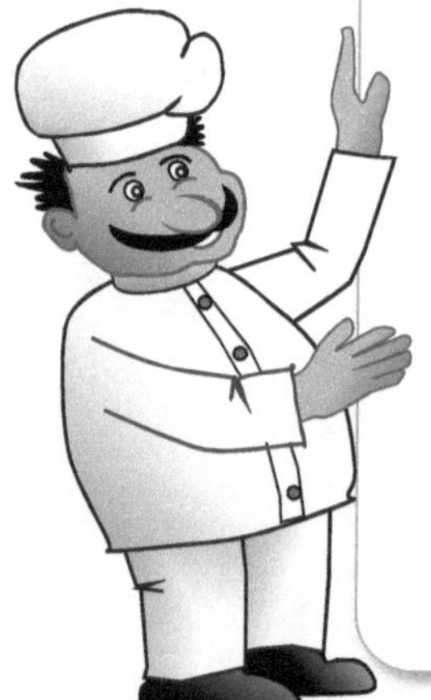

These juices give you
the vitamins, minerals,
antioxidants and
phytochemicals
you need.

All ingredients used
in these juices
must be organic!

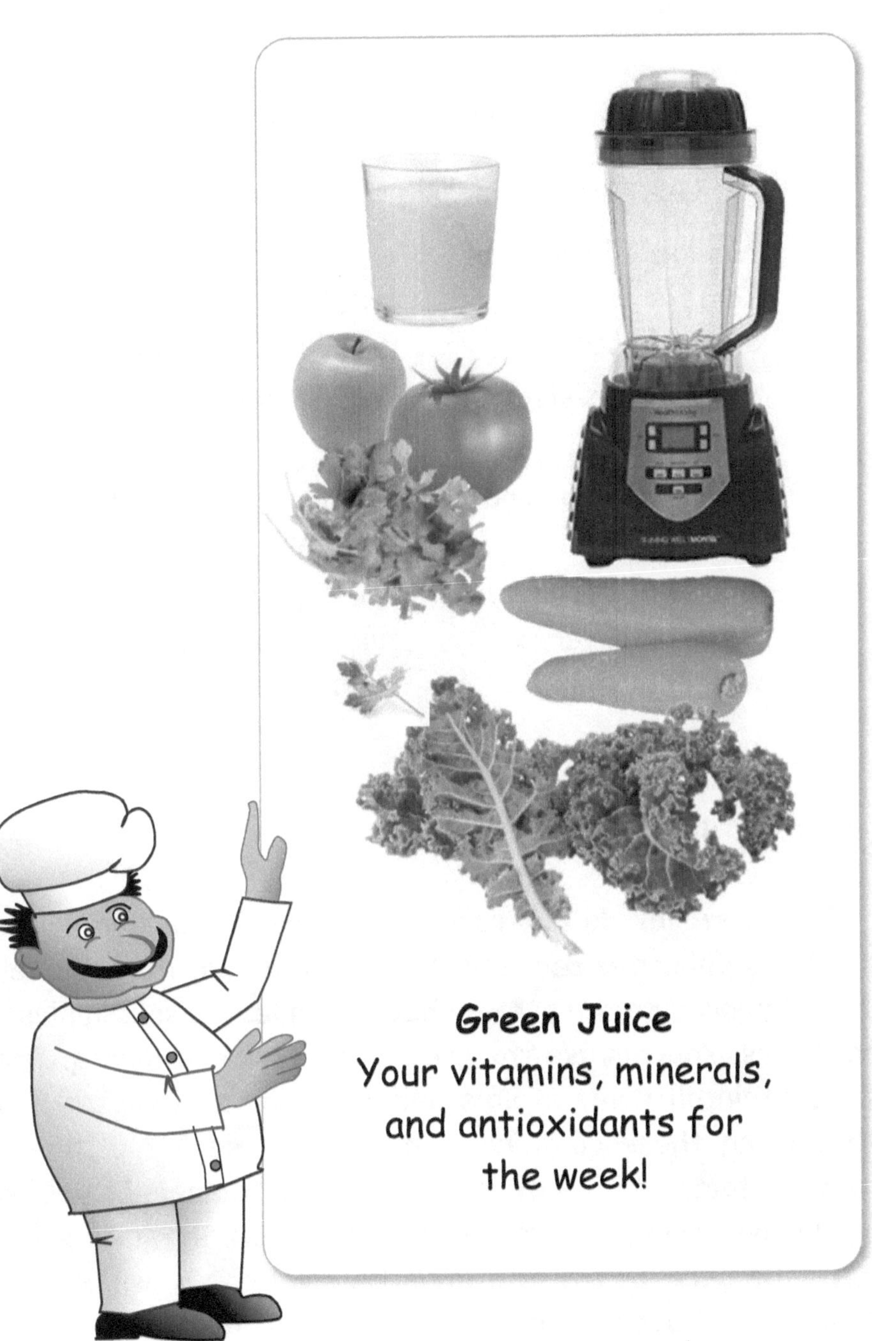

Green Juice
Your vitamins, minerals,
and antioxidants for
the week!

Ingredients

(Makes four large glasses)

Use only organic vegetables and fruits.	
two large leaves* of Kale (or Swiss Chard or Collard Greens)	one apple with skin (preferably not the red delicious apple)
one medium-size red tomato	four sprigs** of cilantro
two medium or one large carrot	six sprigs** of Italian parsley***
one quart (four cups) of filtered water	one cup of orange juice (fresh squeezed or organic from container)
$\frac{1}{2}$-1 cup strawberries	

*Most stores do not carry the large, fresh Kale, Swiss Chard and Collard green leaves. When they do, they are very large compared to the pre-washed green leaves sold in plastic containers. You can use the greens in these containers. They may contain all Kale, or Kale and Spinach, or a variety mix. When using these containers of greens, use 1/2 of the 5-ounce container or 1/4 of the 10-ounce container. If you use green leaves from a container of lettuce mix, the juice will be bitter. Be sure to use the strawberries! They will help to enhance the flavor and remove the "green" taste.

**A sprig is a small stem bearing leaves. See above image for size relationship.

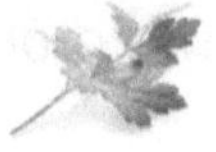

***Do not use parsley if you are pregnant.

Preparation

1. Place all the leafy greens into the high-speed blender/juicer container. (Do not put carrots in first. They may stick under the blades.)

2. Pour in the cup of orange juice.

3. Cut the tomato into quarters and place in container.

4. Remove apple core. Leave skin on. Cut apple into quarters and place in container.

5. Cut carrots into 2- or 3-inch pieces and place in container.

6. Place the strawberries in the container.

7. Add one quart of water.

8. Place lid over container and be sure it is firmly attached.

9. Turn on the blender at low speed and gradually increase to maximum speed. Let it run at high speed for one minute. Be careful not to overfill the container. If it is too full juice may come out and the lid may pop off creating quite a mess to clean up. Packing too much in the container may also overwork the motor in the blender causing it to overheat and stop running.

10. Open lid and remove foam from top of container.

11. The juice is ready to pour and drink!

12. Hold your nose closed when drinking. (Just kidding.)

Notes

If you do not drink all the juice immediately, put it in the refrigerator in a container with a lid. Cold slows down the enzymes in the juice from damaging some of the micro-nutrients. The juice should be consumed the same day. It is not very good the second day.

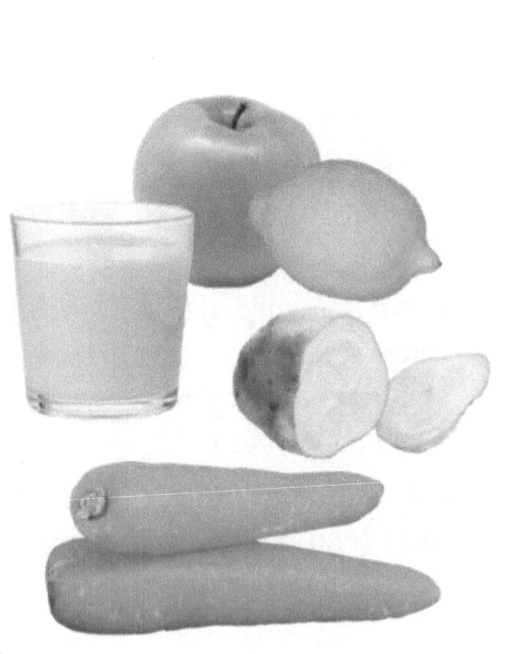

Apple, Carrot & Beet Juice

Your vitamins, minerals and antioxidants for the week!

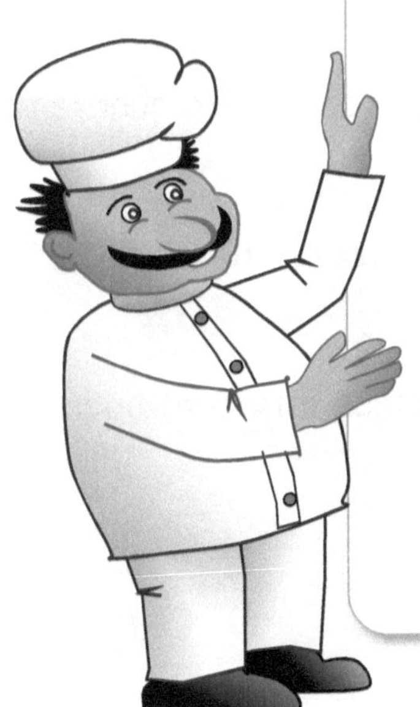

Ingredients
(Makes four large glasses)

Use only organic vegetables and fruits.	
juice squeezed from one lemon (for extra vitamin C)	one quart (four cups) of filtered water
one cup of orange juice (fresh squeezed or organic from container)	one or two apples with skin, preferably not the red delicious apple
one golden or red beet (red beets make a mess)	two medium-large size carrots (or equivalent)

Preparation

1. Remove apple core. Leave skin on. Cut apple into quarters and place in container.

2. Cut carrots into two- or three-inch pieces and place in container.

3. Cut the beet into small pieces and place into container.

4. Pour in the cup of orange juice.

5. Add one quart of water.

6. Place lid over container and be sure it is firmly attached.

7. Turn on the blender at low speed and gradually increase to maximum speed. Let it run at high speed for one minute. Be careful not to overfill the container. If it is too full juice may come out and the lid may pop off creating quite a mess to clean up. Packing too much in the container may also overwork the motor in the blender causing it to overheat and stop running.

8. Open lid and remove foam from top of container.

9. The Juice is ready to pour and drink!

Notes

If you do not drink all the juice immediately, put it in the refrigerator in a container with a lid. Cold slows down the enzymes in the juice from damaging some of the micro-nutrients. The juice should be consumed the same day. It is not very good the second day.

Organic Fast-Food Recipes

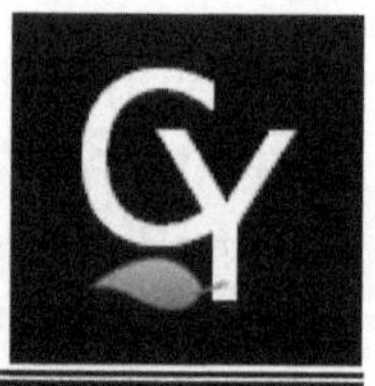

Quick, Easy and Inexpensive Meals
With 3 to 5 Ingredients

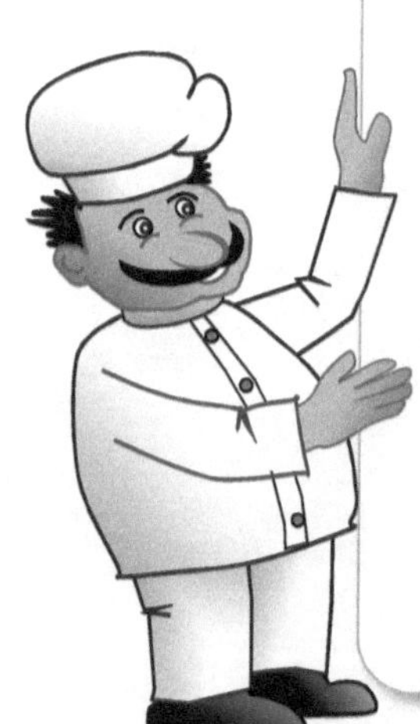

Organic Fast-Food Recipes

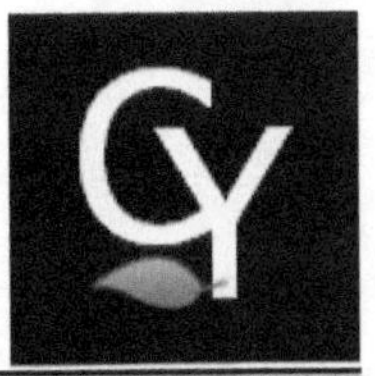

Quick, Easy and Inexpensive Meals
With 3 to 5 Ingredients

The following meals are not perfect, but they are far better than the standard American diet (SAD).

These organic fast-food recipes are meant to serve as a transition from an unhealthy SAD diet to a healthy organic, plant-based diet.

You should drink one or two of the juices each week to be sure you are getting the essential micronutrients.

Organic Fast-Food Recipes

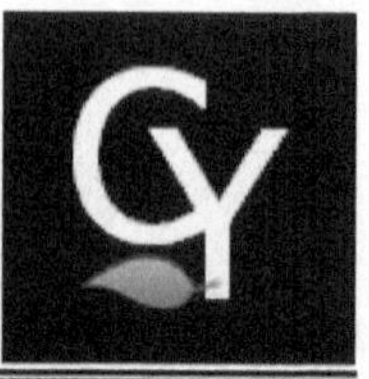

Quick, Easy and Inexpensive Meals
With 3 to 5 Ingredients

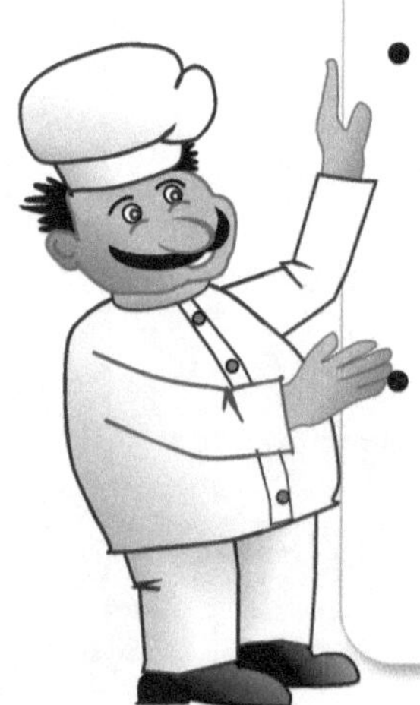

TIPS FOR QUICK & TASTY PREPARATION

- Use a small amount of quality sesame oil or olive oil in the pan for frying and sautéing.
- Use a microwave or toaster oven to save time.
- Use a small amount of water in a pan to cook and steam potato chunks and other vegetables.
- Microwave potatoes and meat substitutes before baking in toaster oven.

*Making your switch
to a healthier diet
much easier!*

MEATBALL HOAGIE & STEAK FRIES or CHIPS

1. gardein organic meatball substitute

2. hoagie bun toasted

3. Newman's organic marinara sauce

4. organic steak cut fries or lightly salted potato chips

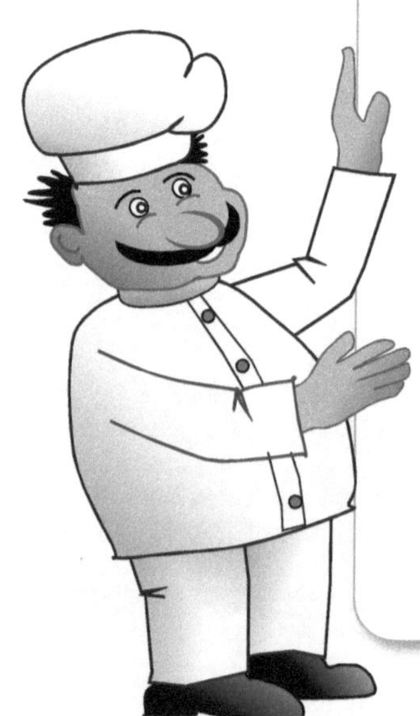

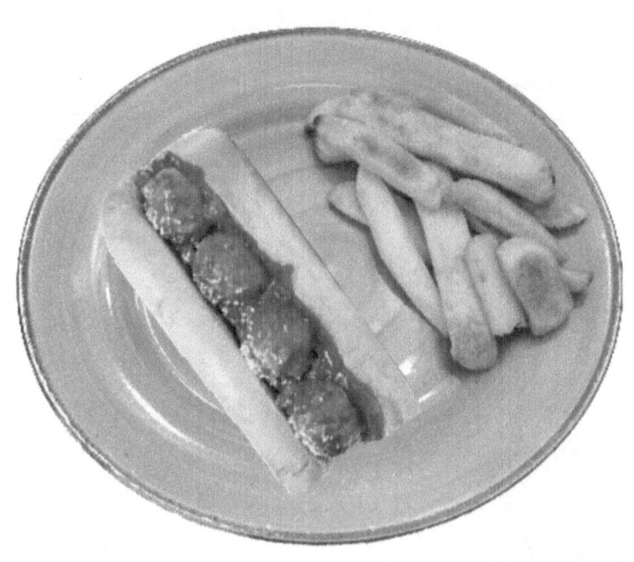

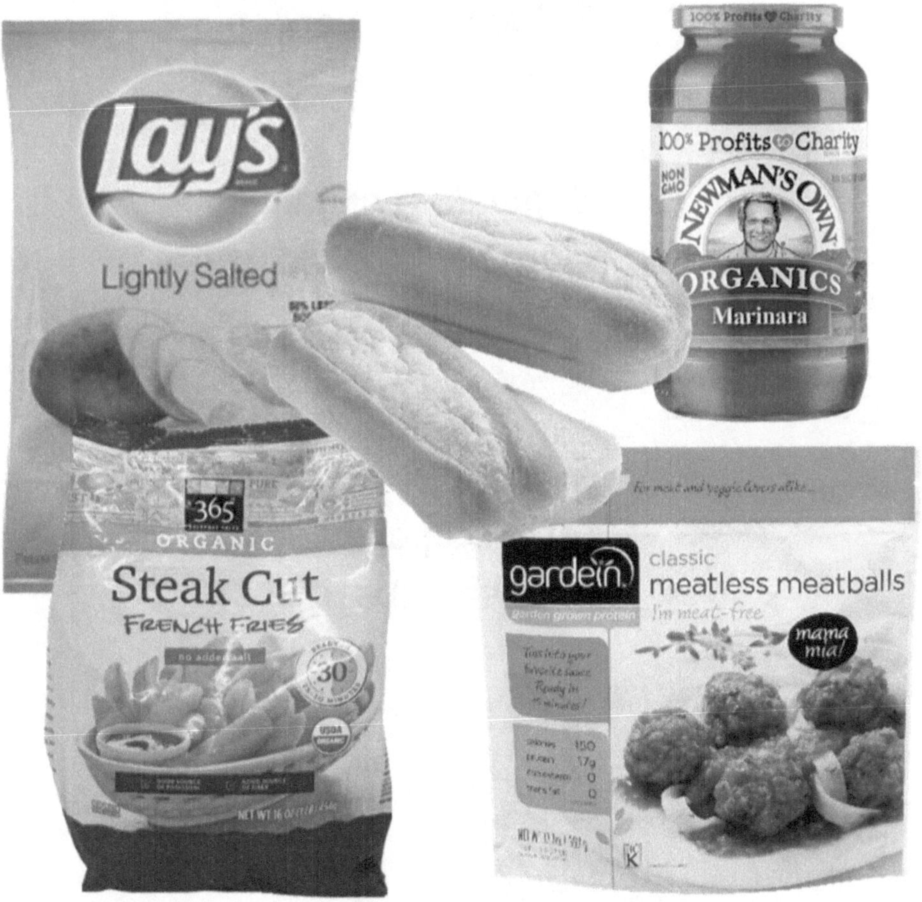

Lay's
Lightly Salted
100% Profits Charity
NON GMO
NEWMAN'S OWN
ORGANICS
Marinara
365
ORGANIC
Steak Cut
FRENCH FRIES
30
gardein
classic
meatless meatballs
I'm meat-free
mama mia!

SPAGHETTI & MEATBALLS

1. organic spaghetti noodles

2. Newman's organic marinara sauce

3. gardein organic meatball substitute

ADD CHEESE

4. nutritional yeast (grated parmesan cheese substitute)

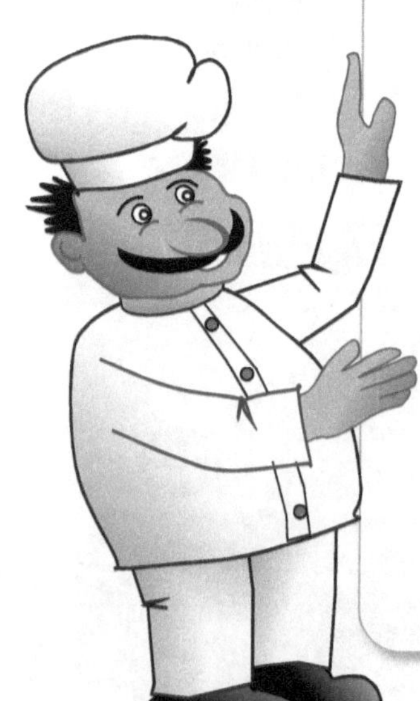

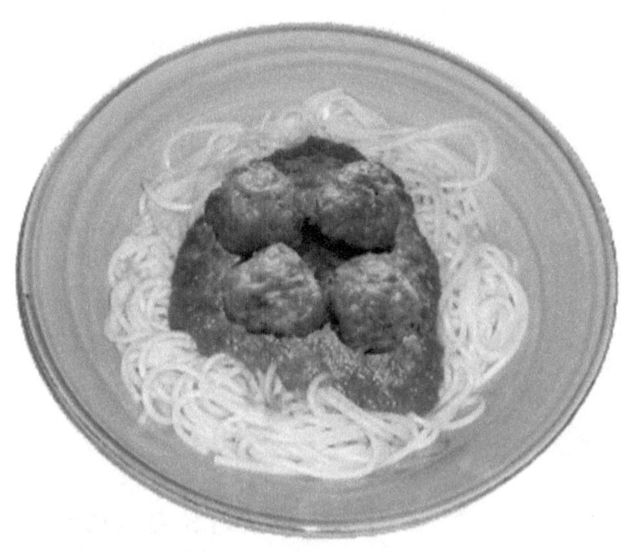

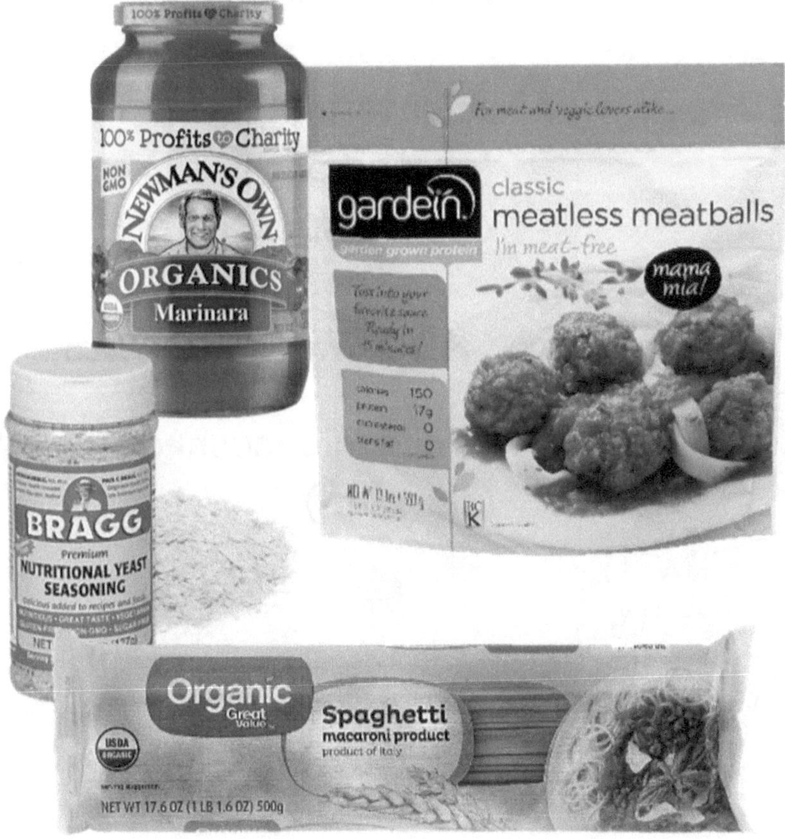
100% Profits to Charity
NON GMO
NEWMAN'S OWN
ORGANICS
Marinara
BRAGG
Premium
NUTRITIONAL YEAST
SEASONING
For meat and veggie lovers alike...
gardein.
garden grown protein
classic
meatless meatballs
I'm meat-free
mama mia!
Organic
Great Value
Spaghetti
macaroni product
product of Italy
USDA ORGANIC
NET WT 17.6 OZ (1 LB 1.6 OZ) 500g

SPAGHETTI

1. organic spaghetti noodles

2. Newman's organic marinara sauce

3. nutritional yeast (grated parmesan cheese substitute)

ADD MUSHROOMS

4. organic mushrooms (sautéed)

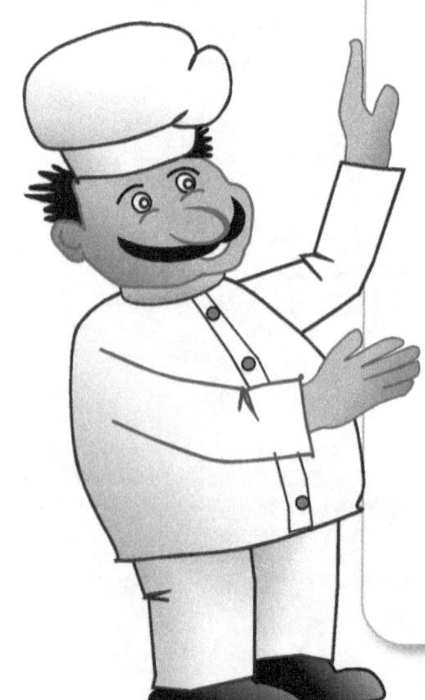

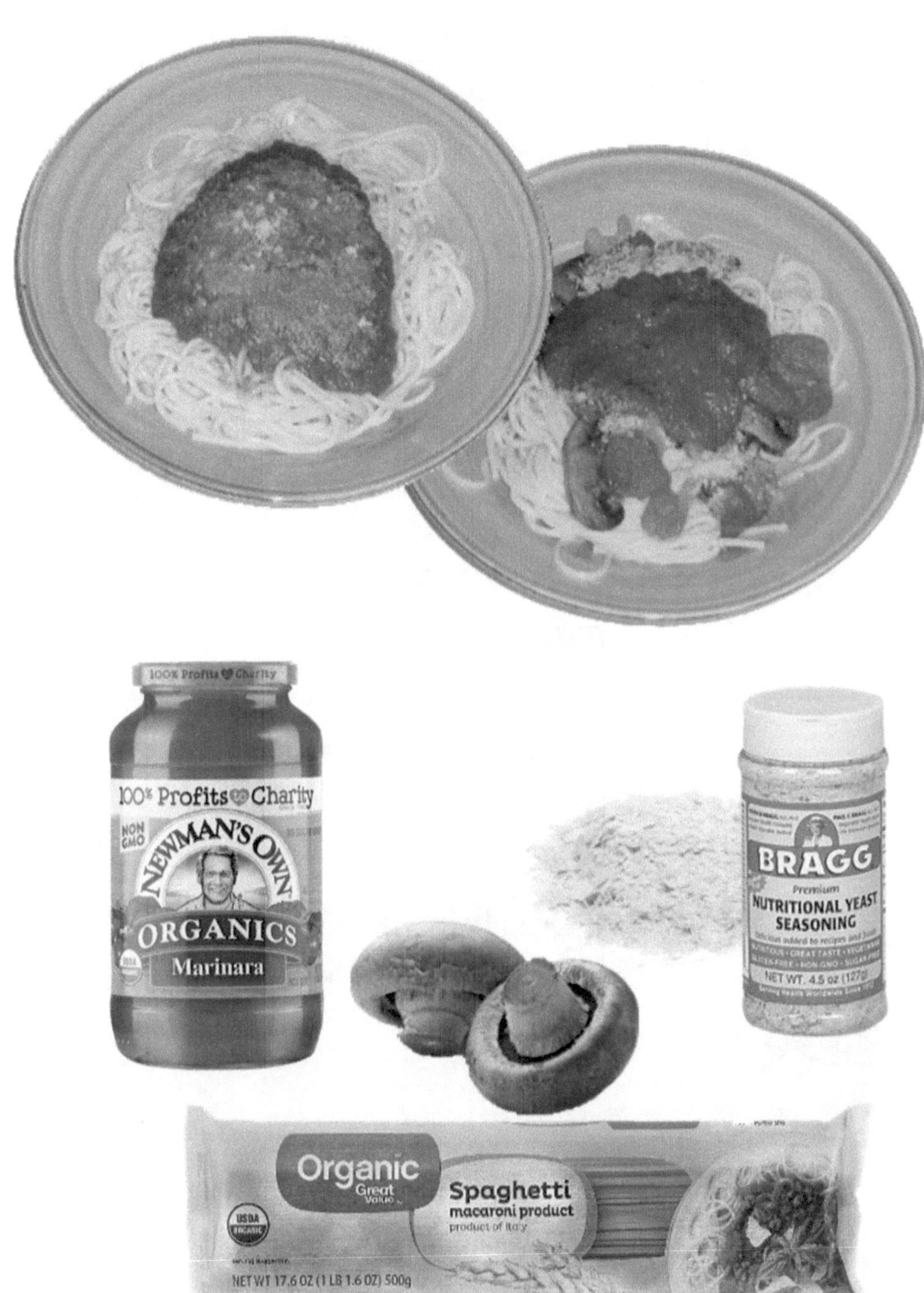

100% Profits Charity
NON GMO
NEWMAN'S OWN
ORGANICS
Marinara
BRAGG
Premium
NUTRITIONAL YEAST
SEASONING
NET WT. 4.5 oz (127g)
Organic
Great Value
Spaghetti
macaroni product
product of Italy
USDA ORGANIC
NET WT 17.6 OZ (1 LB 1.6 OZ) 500g

SPAGHETTI & GREEN BEANS

1. organic spaghetti noodles

2. Newman's organic marinara sauce

3. organic green beans

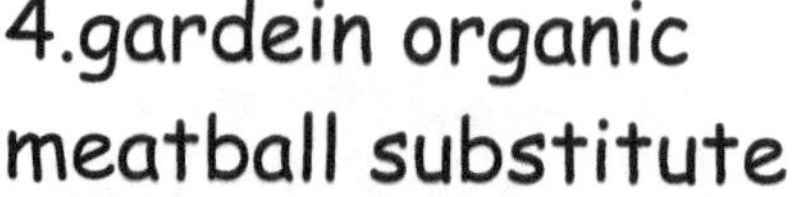

4.gardein organic meatball substitute

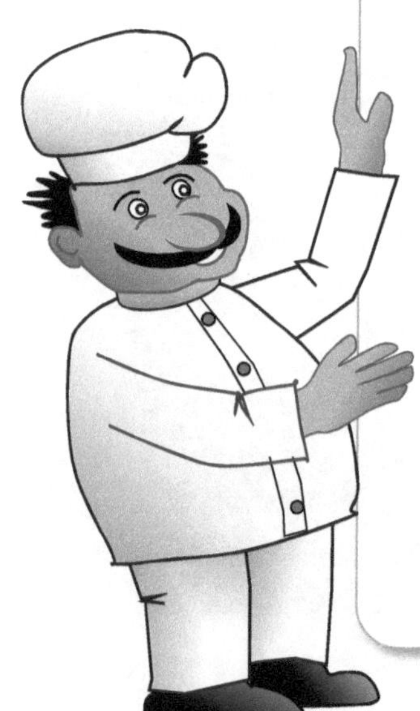

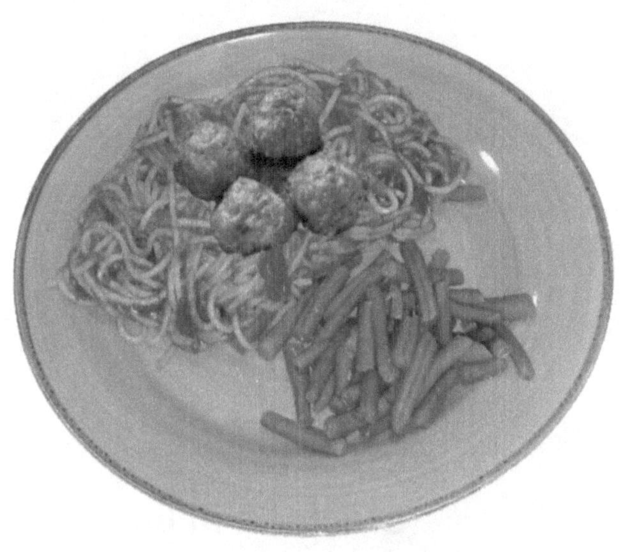

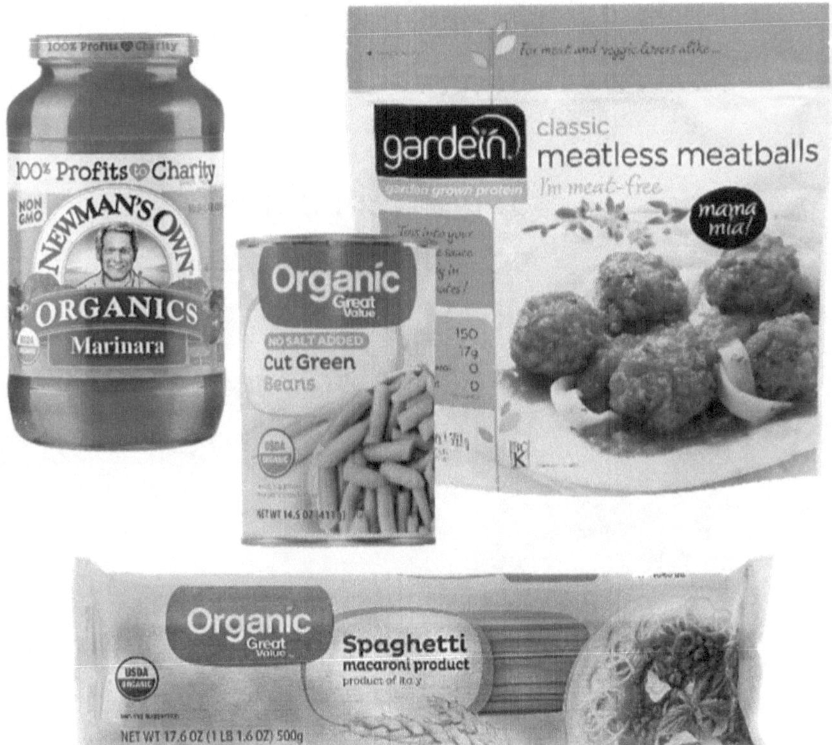
100% Profits Charity
NON GMO
NEWMAN'S OWN
ORGANICS
Marinara

Organic
Great Value
NO SALT ADDED
Cut Green
Beans
USDA ORGANIC
NET WT 14.5 OZ (411 g)

for meat and veggie lovers alike...
gardein
garden grown protein
classic
meatless meatballs
I'm meat-free
mama mia!
150
17g
0
0

Organic
Great Value
USDA ORGANIC
Spaghetti
macaroni product
product of Italy
NET WT 17.6 OZ (1 LB 1.6 OZ) 500g

CHICKEN, POTATO & BEANS

1. organic
red potatoes
(steamed in pan)

2. organic green
beans

3. gardein chicken
scallopini substitute

4. earth balance
butter substitute

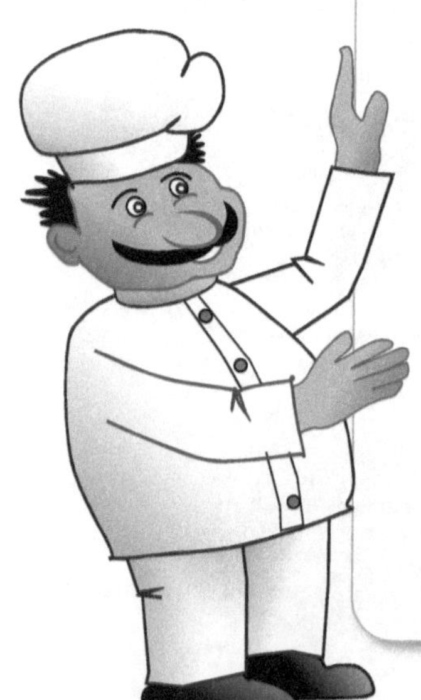

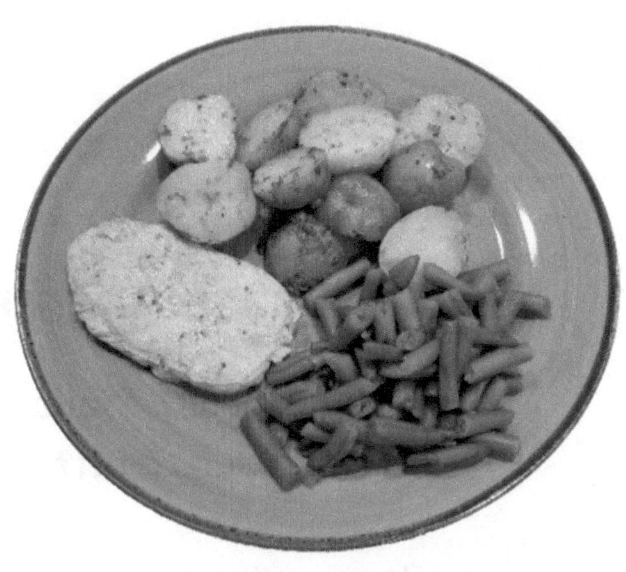

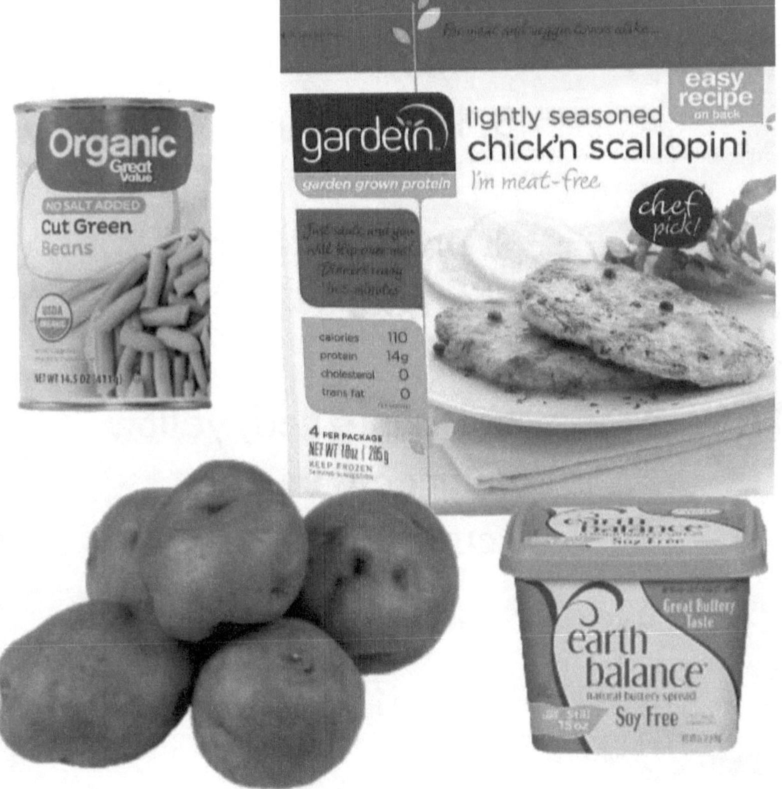
Organic
Great Value
NO SALT ADDED
Cut Green
Beans
USDA
NET WT 14.5 OZ (411g)
gardein
garden grown protein
lightly seasoned
chick'n scallopini
I'm meat-free
easy
recipe
on back
chef
pick!
calories 110
protein 14g
cholesterol 0
trans fat 0
4 PER PACKAGE
NET WT 10oz (285 g)
KEEP FROZEN
earth
balance
natural buttery spread
Soy Free
Great Buttery
Taste

ITALIAN
SAUSAGE HOAGIE

1. Field Roast Italian sausage substitute

2. organic steak cut fries

3. hoagie bun toasted

4. organic onion, sautéed

5.organic red, yellow or green pepper sautéed

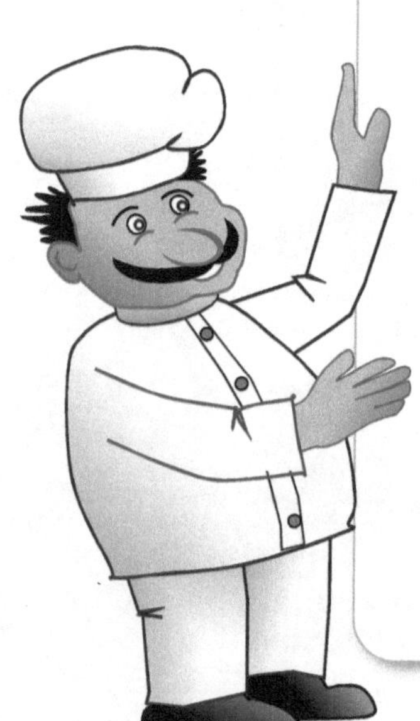

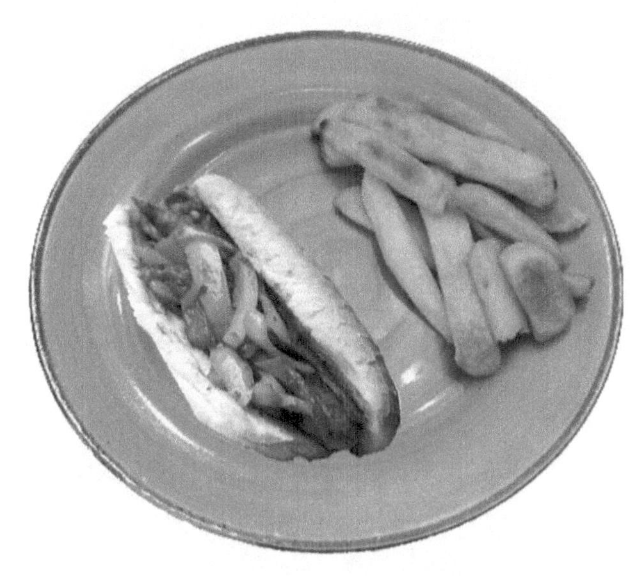

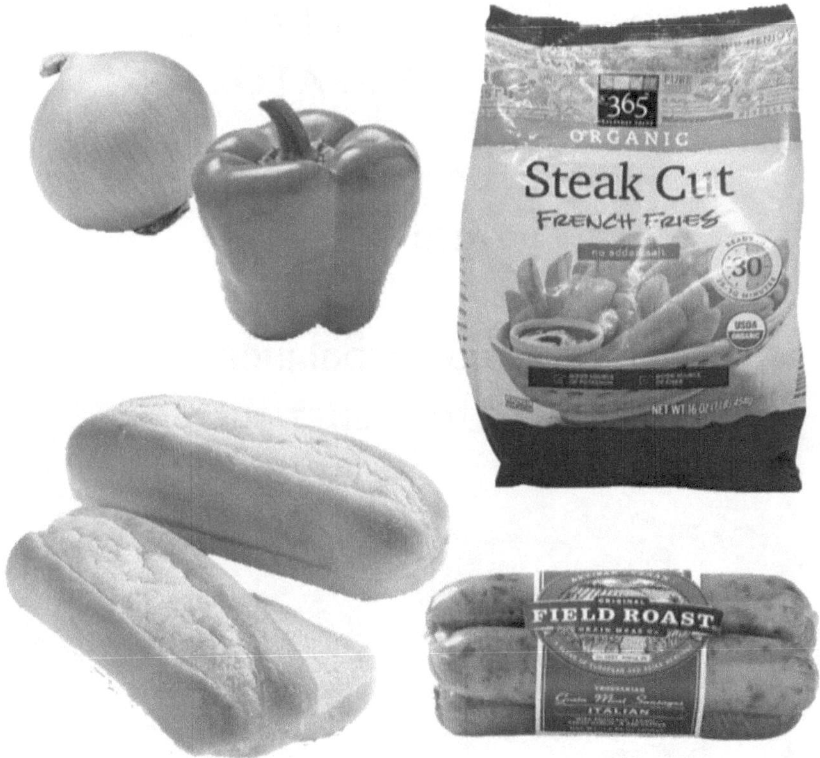
365
ORGANIC
Steak Cut
FRENCH FRIES
no added salt
30
USDA
ORGANIC
NET WT 16 OZ (1 LB) 454g
ORIGINAL
FIELD ROAST
GRAIN MEAT CO.
VEGETARIAN
Grain Meat Sausages
ITALIAN

CHILI & CHIPS

1. Amy's organic chili

2. organic blue corn chips

ADD A BAKED POTATO

3. organic Russet potato

4. earth balance butter substitute

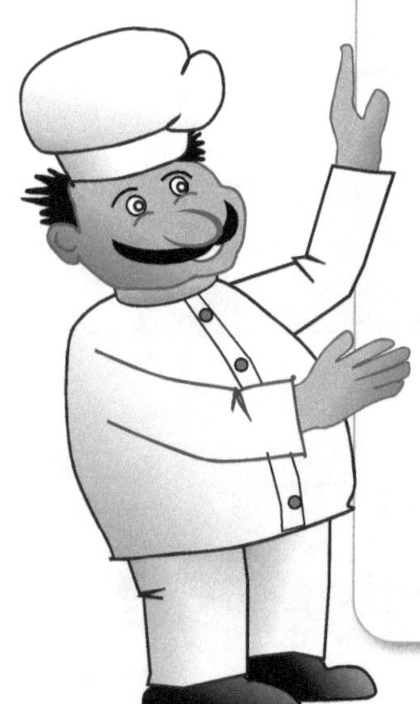

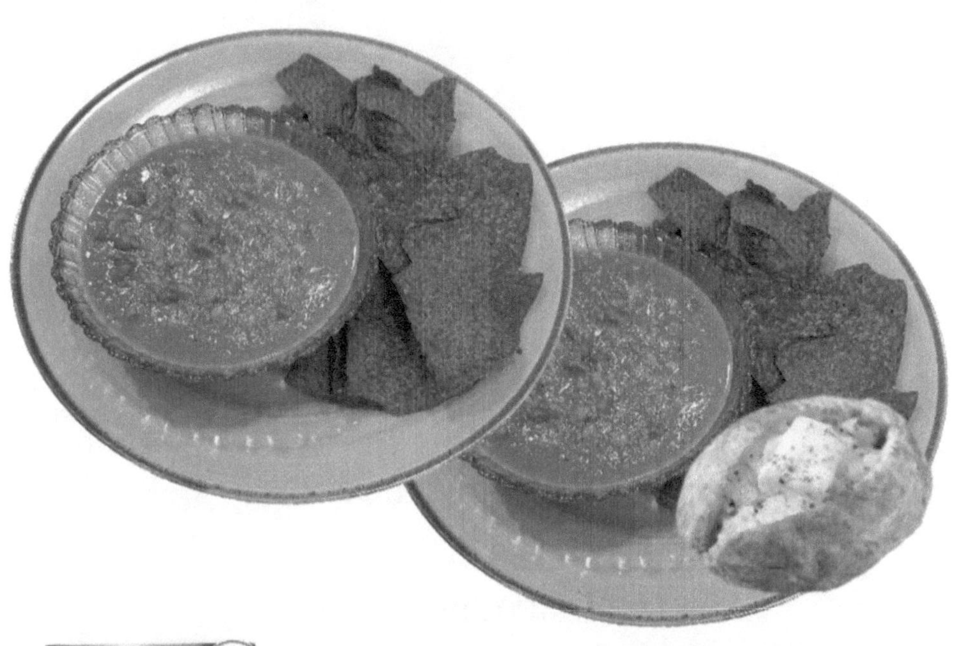

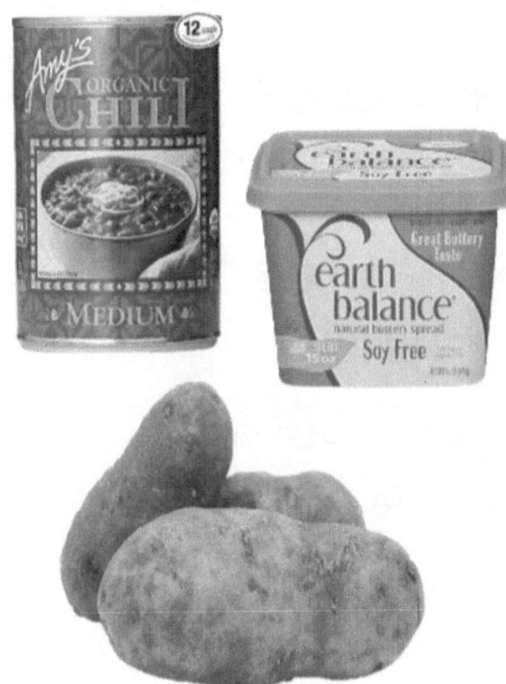
Amy's
ORGANIC
CHILI
MEDIUM
earth
balance
natural buttery spread
Soy Free
Great Buttery
Taste

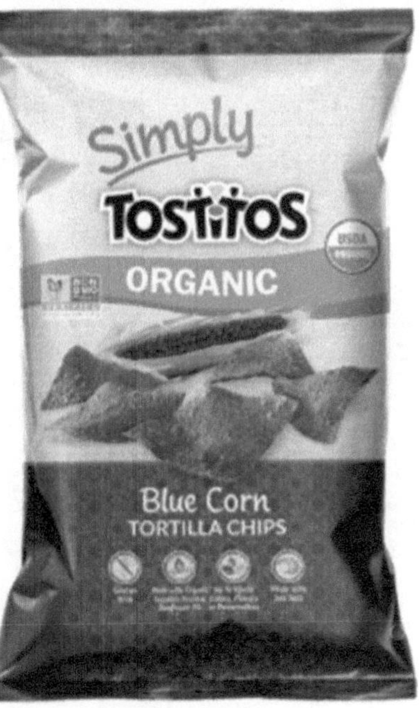
Simply
TOSTITOS
ORGANIC
Blue Corn
TORTILLA CHIPS

MASHED POTATOES & PEAS

1. organic Yukon
gold potatoes

2. organic peas

3. earth balance
butter substitute

ADD RED PEPPER HUMMUS

4. organic roasted
red pepper hummus

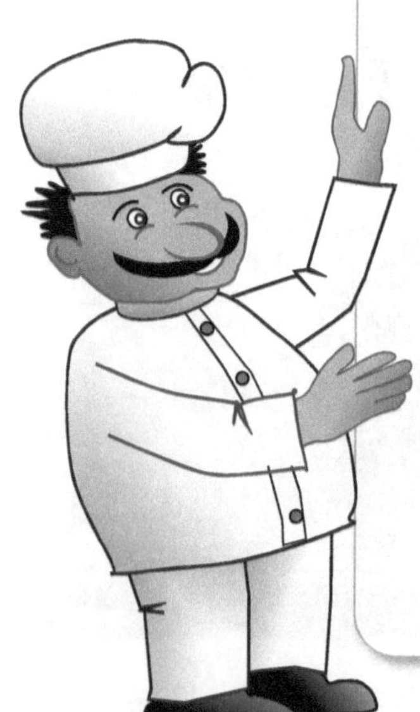

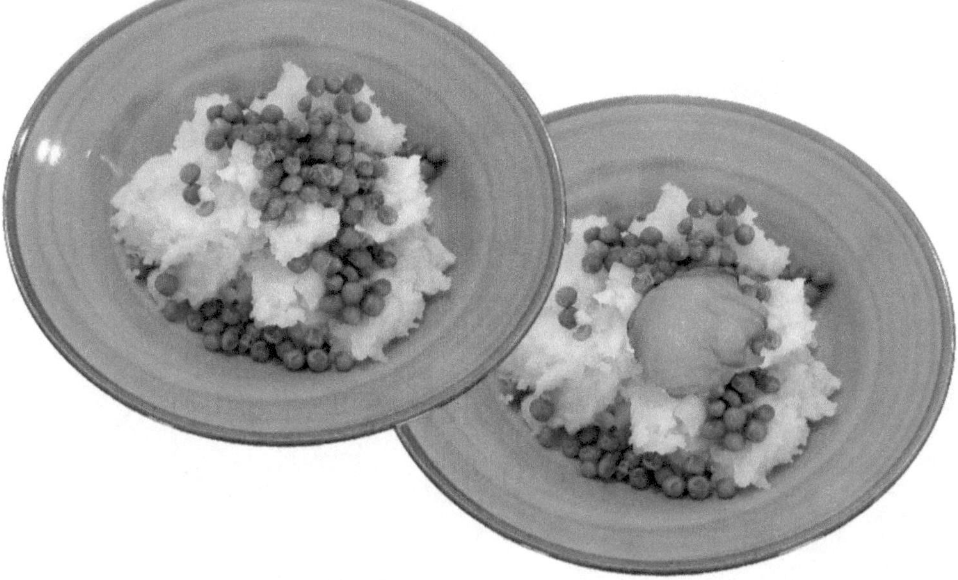

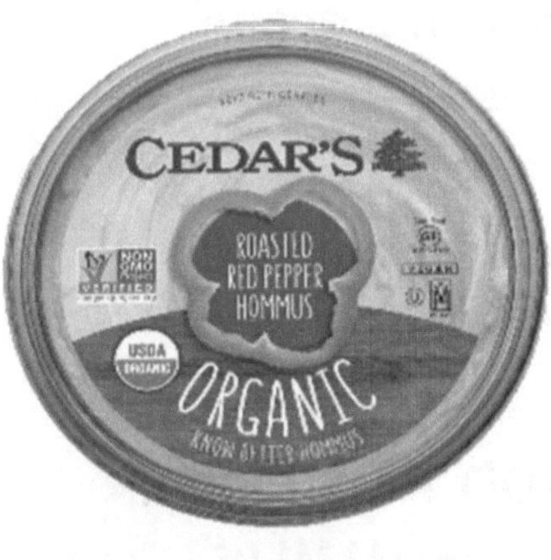

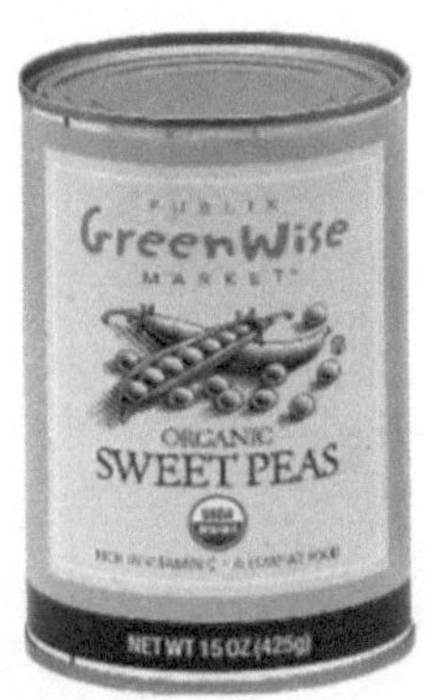

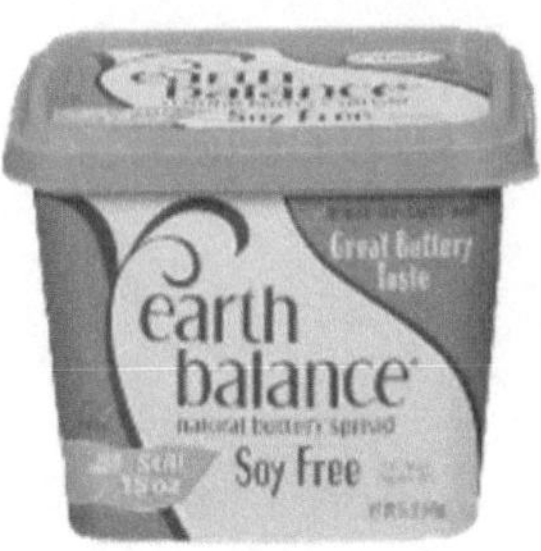

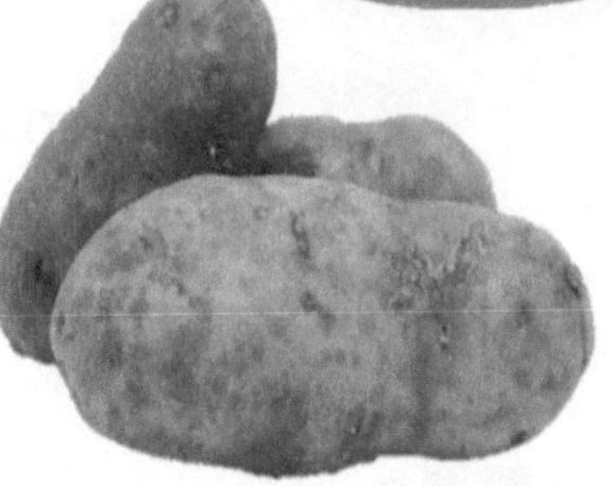

MASHED POTATOES & GREEN BEANS

1. organic Yukon gold potatoes

2. organic green beans

3. earth balance butter substitute

ADD RED PEPPER HUMMUS

4. organic red pepper hummus

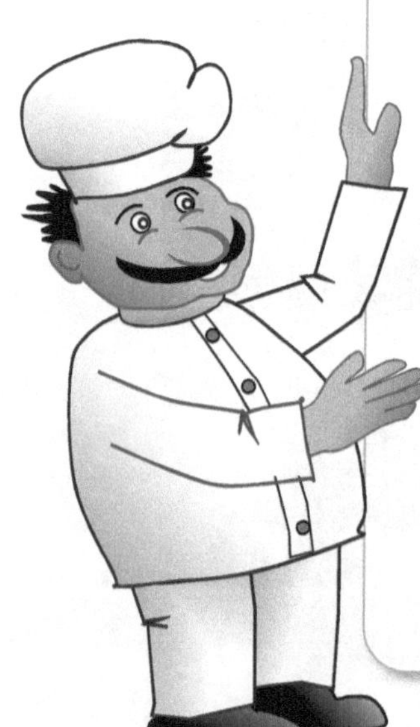

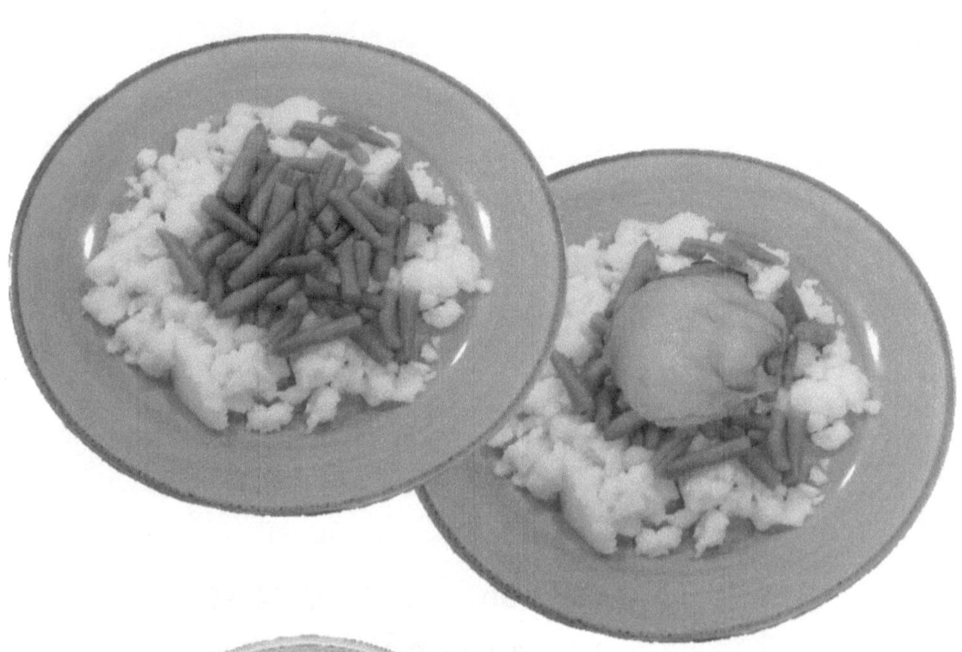

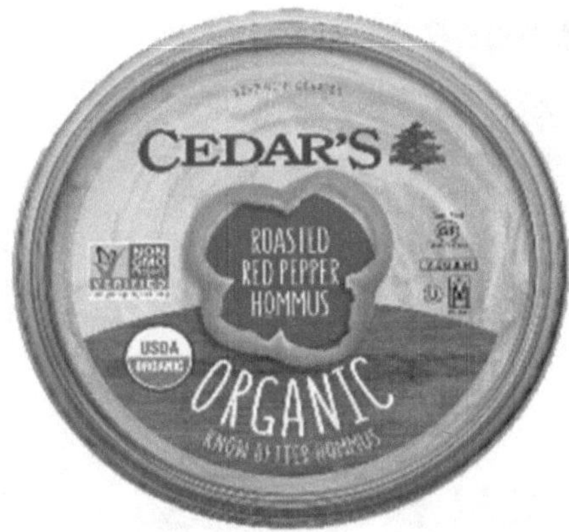
CEDAR'S
ROASTED
RED PEPPER
HOMMUS
USDA
ORGANIC
ORGANIC
KNOW BETTER HOMMUS

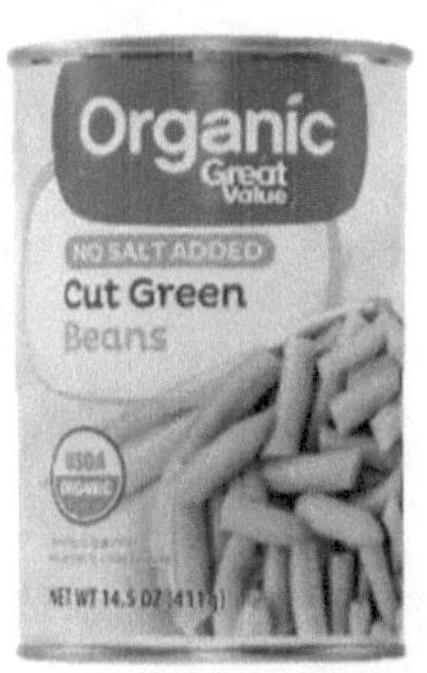
Organic
Great
Value
NO SALT ADDED
Cut Green
Beans
USDA
ORGANIC
NET WT 14.5 OZ (411 g)

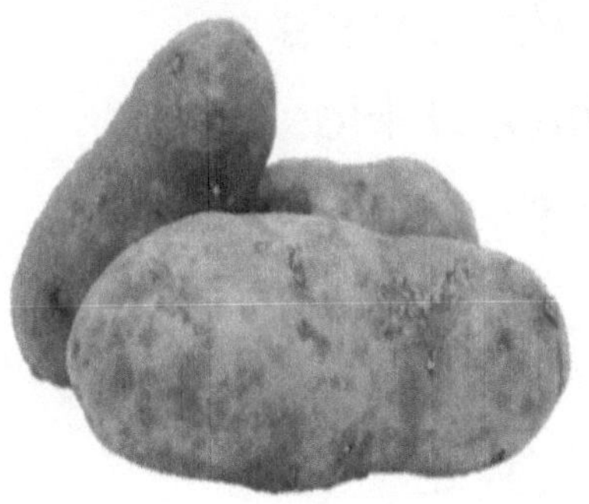

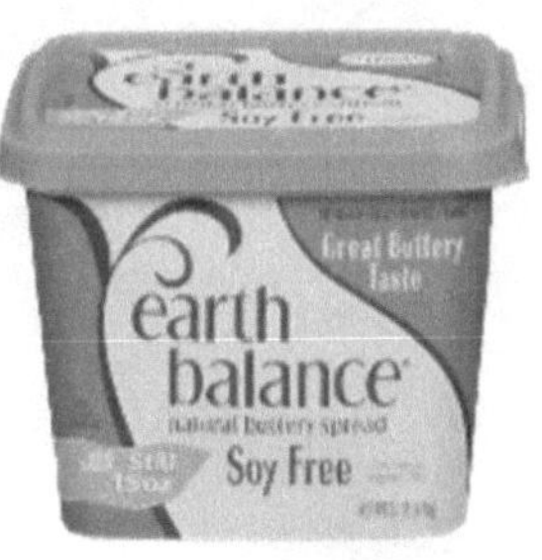
earth
balance
Soy Free
Great Buttery
Taste
earth
balance
natural buttery spread
Soy Free

PANCAKES & SAUSAGE LINKS

1. Birch Benders non-dairy organic pancakes

2. Field Roast smoked apple sage sausage links substitute

3. organic maple syrup

ADD HASH BROWNS

4. dr. Praeger's Southwest Hash Browns

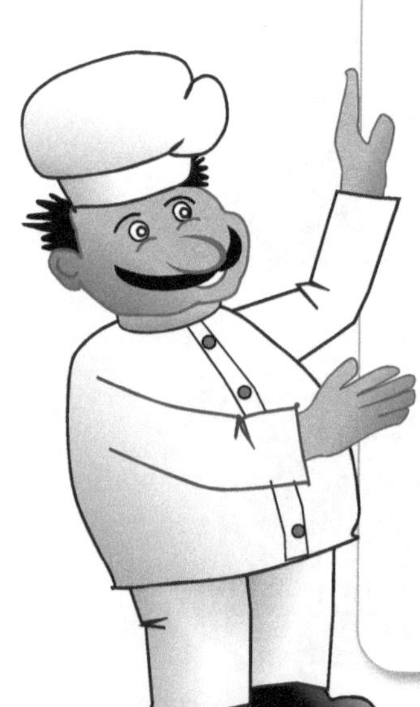

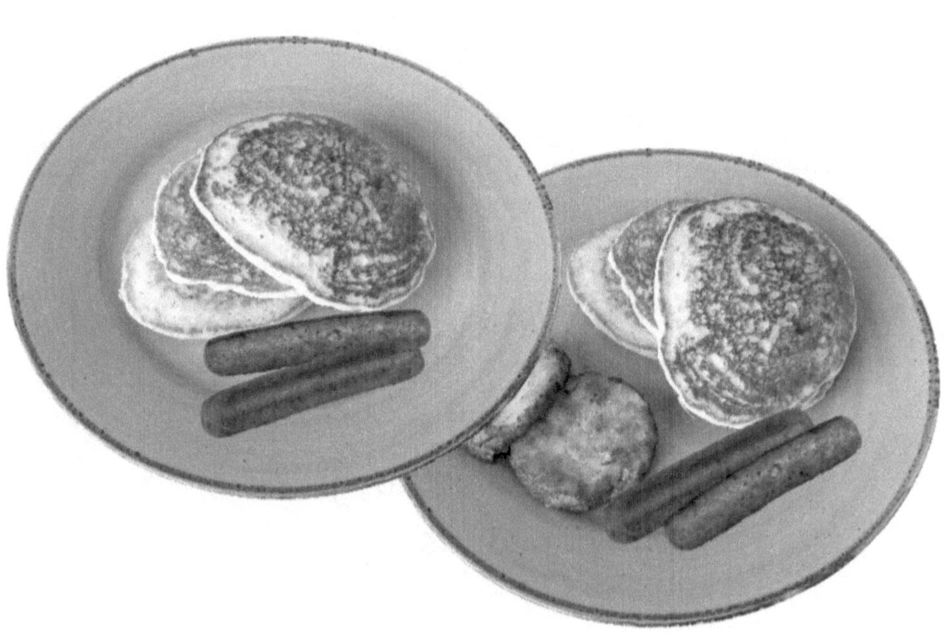

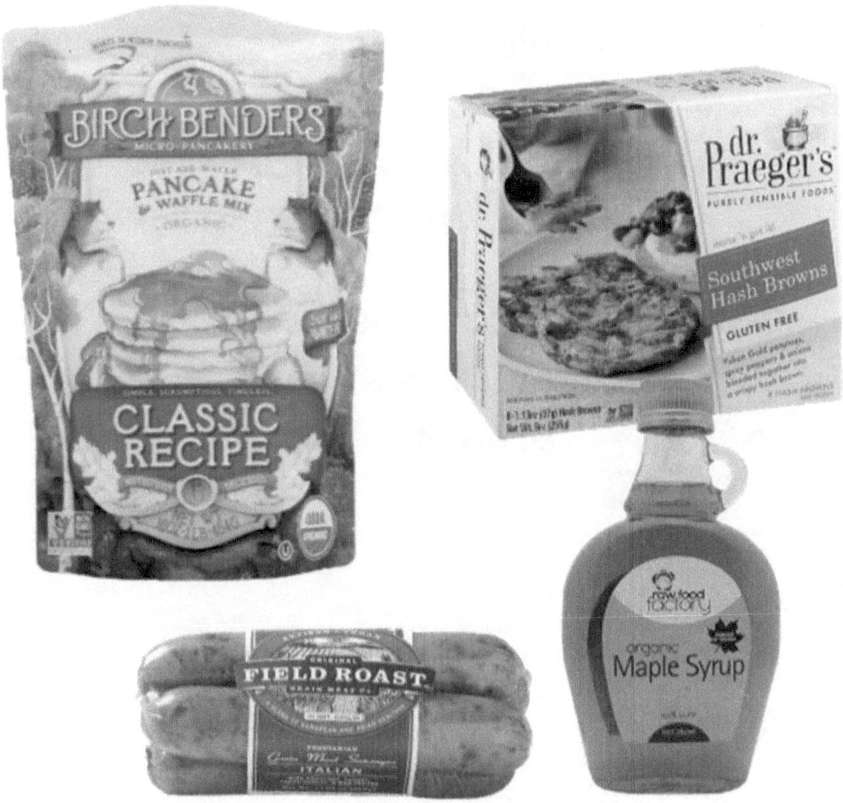

PANCAKES & BLUEBERRIES

1. Birch Benders non-dairy organic pancakes

2. fresh organic blueberries

ADD HASH BROWNS

3. dr. Praeger's Southwest Hash Browns

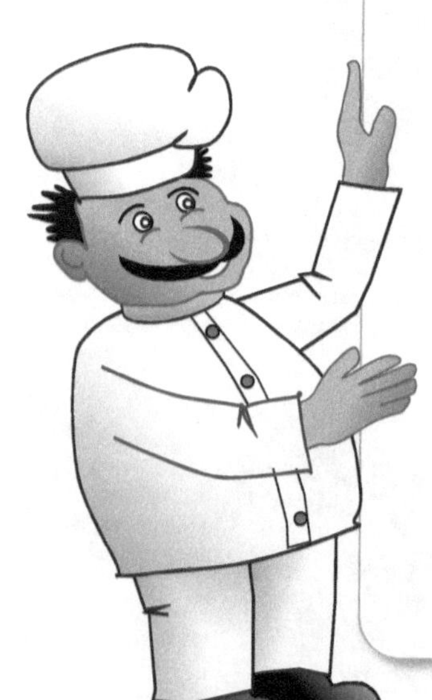

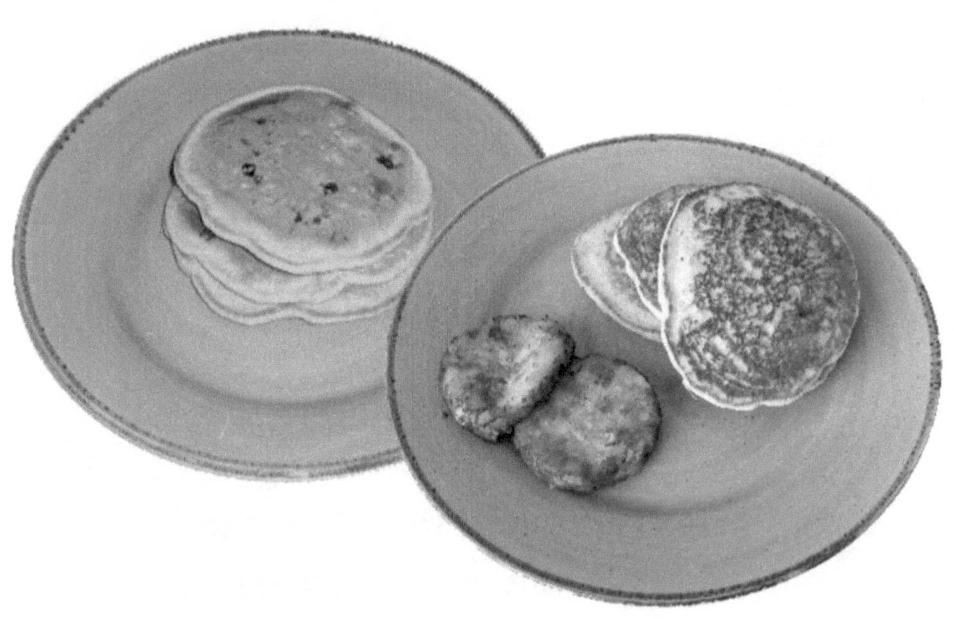

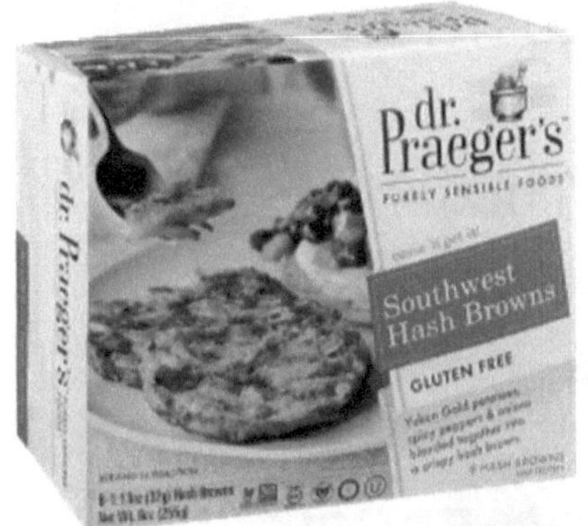

dr.
Praeger's
PURELY SENSIBLE FOODS
Southwest
Hash Browns
GLUTEN FREE

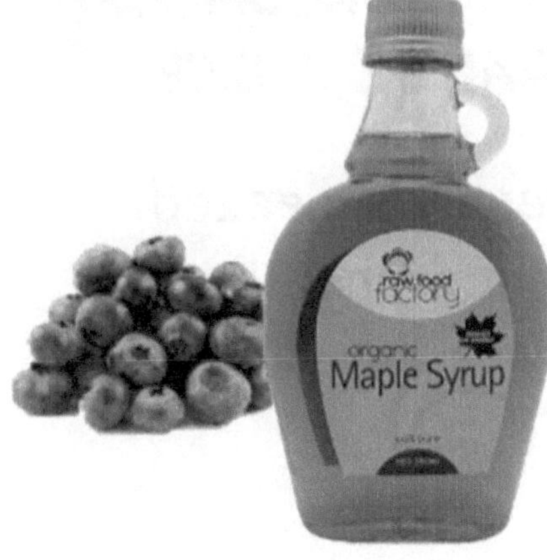

organic
Maple Syrup

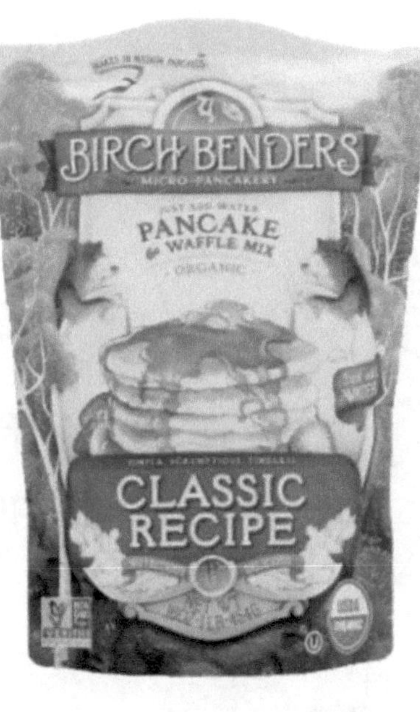

BIRCH BENDERS
MICRO-PANCAKERY
PANCAKE
& WAFFLE MIX
ORGANIC
CLASSIC
RECIPE

EGGS, SAUSAGE, HASH BROWNS

1. organic eggs

2. Field Roast smoked apple sage sausage links substitute

3. dr. Praeger's Southwest Hash Browns

ADD FRESH ORANGE JUICE

4. freshly squeezed organic orange juice

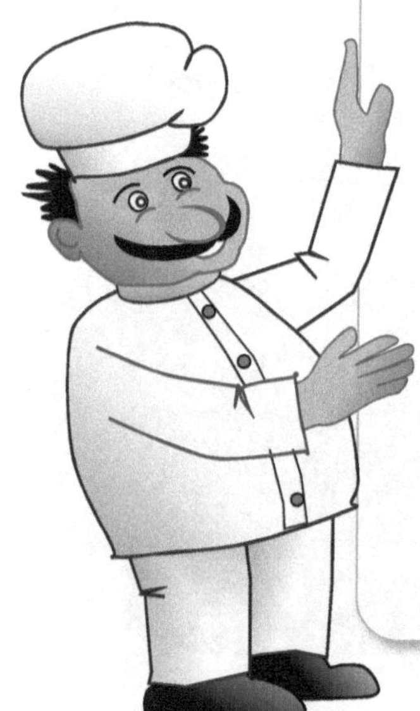

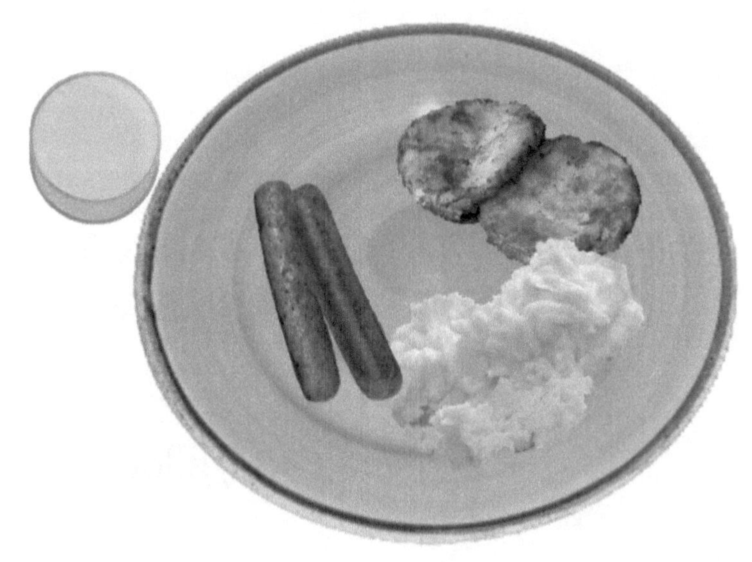

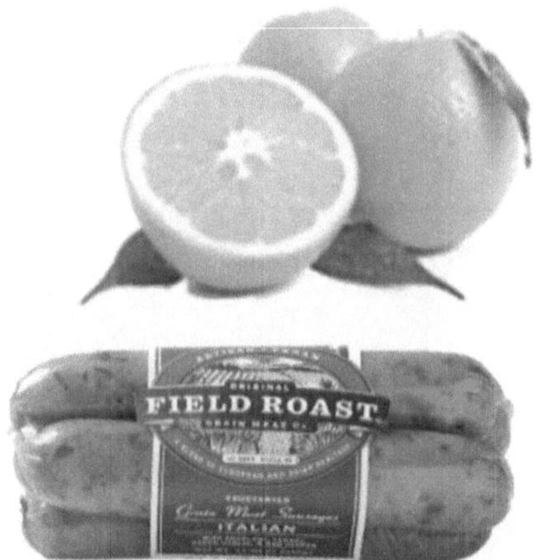
FIELD ROAST
ORIGINAL
GRAIN MEAT Co.
ITALIAN

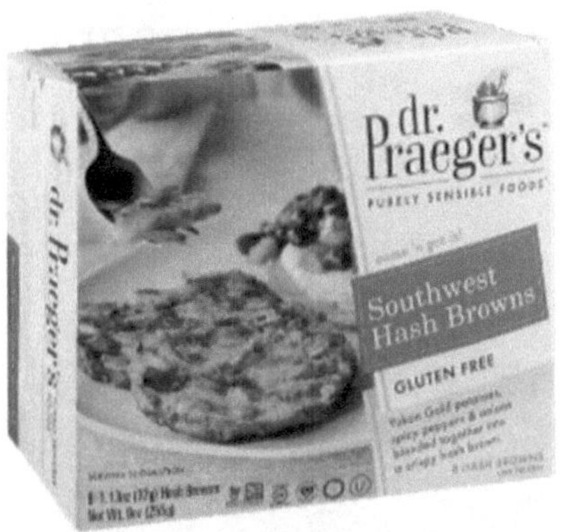
dr.
Praeger's
PURELY SENSIBLE FOODS
Southwest
Hash Browns
GLUTEN FREE

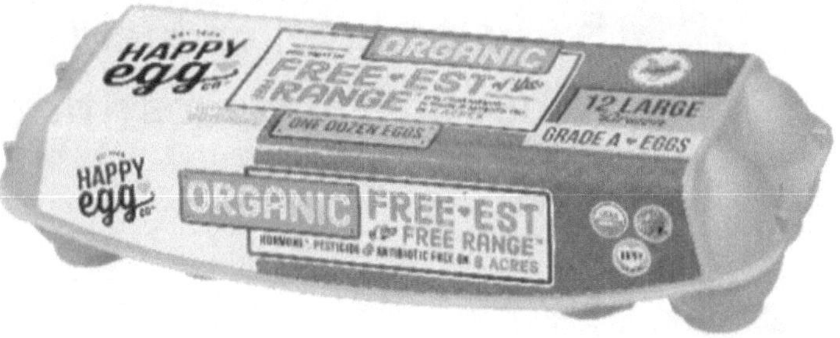
HAPPY
egg co.
ORGANIC
FREE-EST of the
RANGE
ONE DOZEN EGGS
12 LARGE
GRADE A EGGS
HAPPY
egg co.
ORGANIC FREE-EST
of the FREE RANGE
HORMONE, PESTICIDE & ANTIBIOTIC FREE ON 8 ACRES

POTATOES, CARROTS, RED PEPPERS, BEETS & SAUSAGE

1. organic red/yellow potatoes

2. organic red or green pepper

3. organic carrots

4.organic golden beets
(steam 1-4 in same pan)

5.Gimme Lean or Field Roast sausage substitute

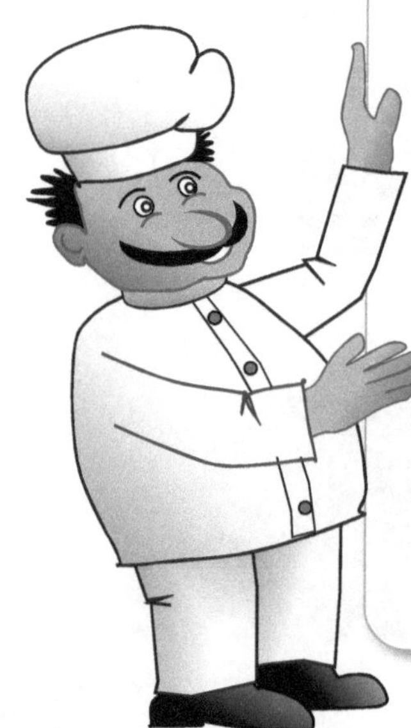

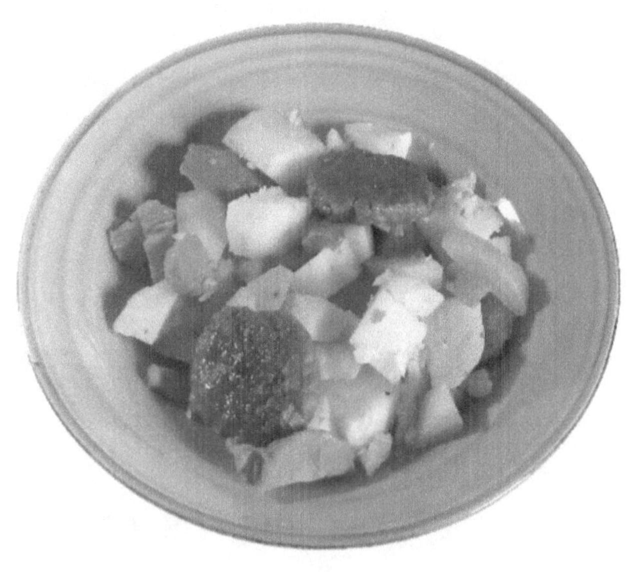

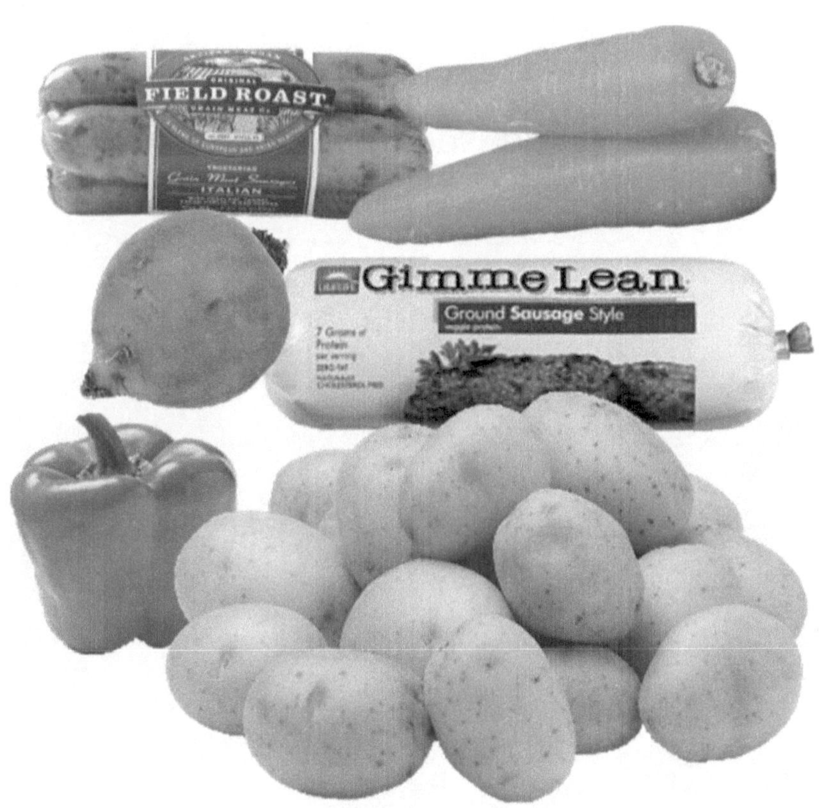
ORIGINAL
FIELD ROAST
GRAIN MEAT CO.
ITALIAN
GimmeLean
Ground Sausage Style
7 Grams of
Protein

MASHED POTATOES, SAUSAGE & GREEN BEANS

1. organic russet potatoes

2. Gimme Lean sausage patties substitute

3. organic green beans

4. earth balance butter substitute

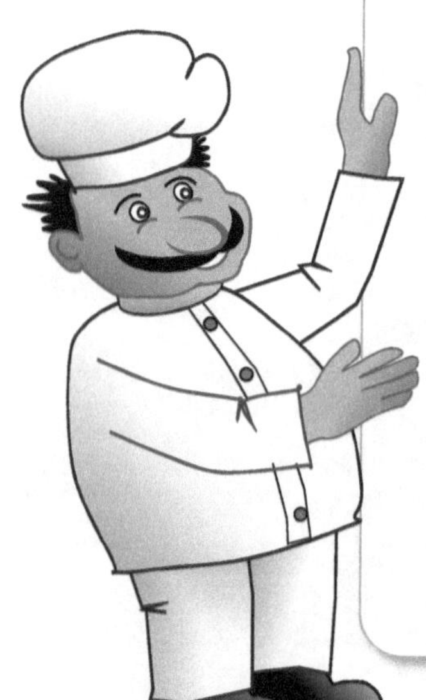

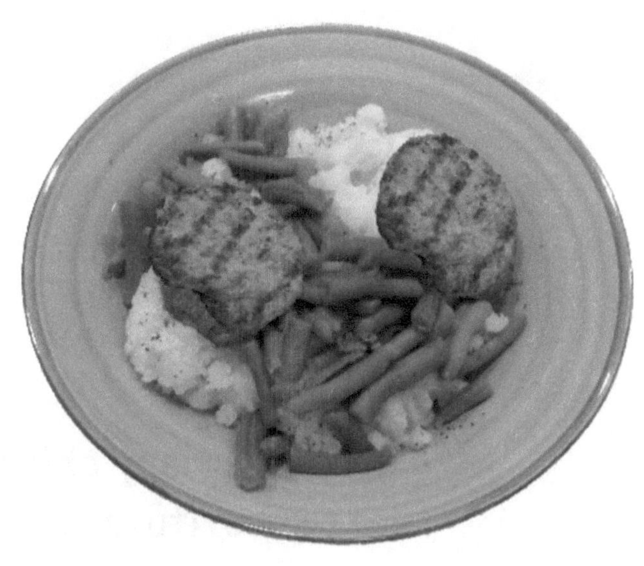

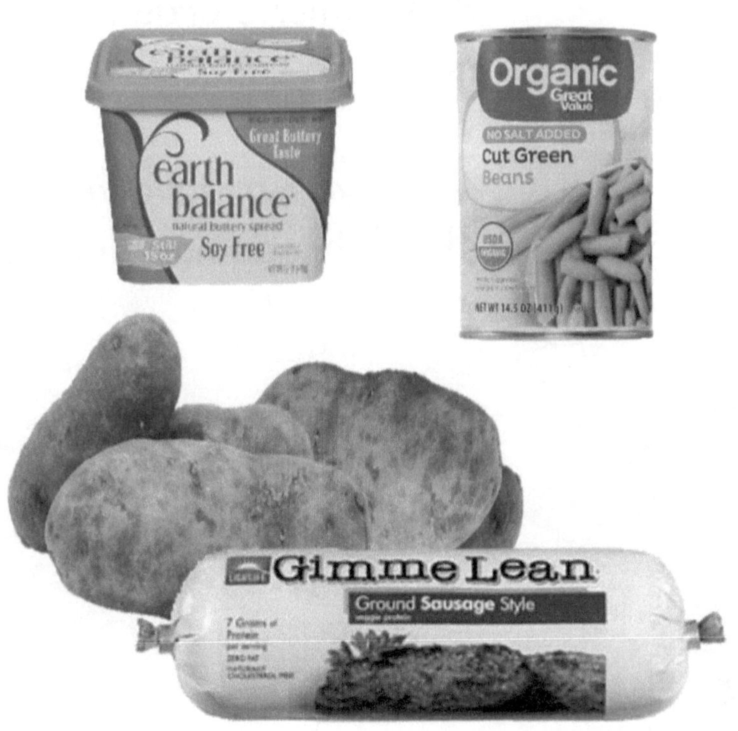

Great Buttery Taste
earth balance
natural buttery spread
Soy Free
Organic
Great Value
NO SALT ADDED
Cut Green Beans
USDA ORGANIC
NET WT 14.5 OZ (411g)
Gimme Lean
Ground Sausage Style
7 Grams of Protein
ZERO FAT
CHOLESTEROL FREE

CHICKEN PARMESAN

1. organic spaghetti noodles
2.gardein crispy chick'n filets substitute

3. Newman's organic marinara sauce

4. daiya mozzarella style shreds non-dairy

ADD MUSHROOMS

5. organic mushrooms (sautéed)

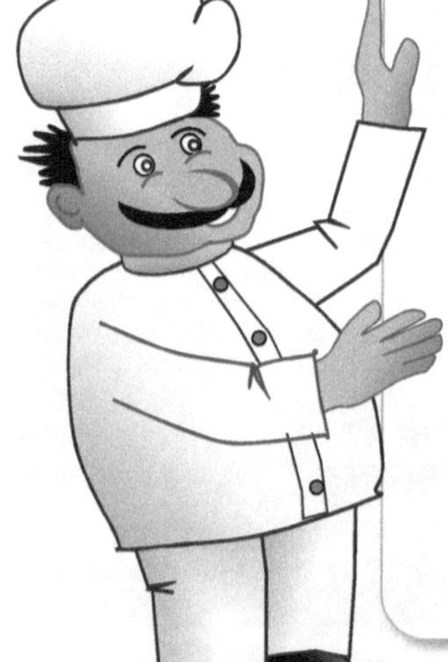

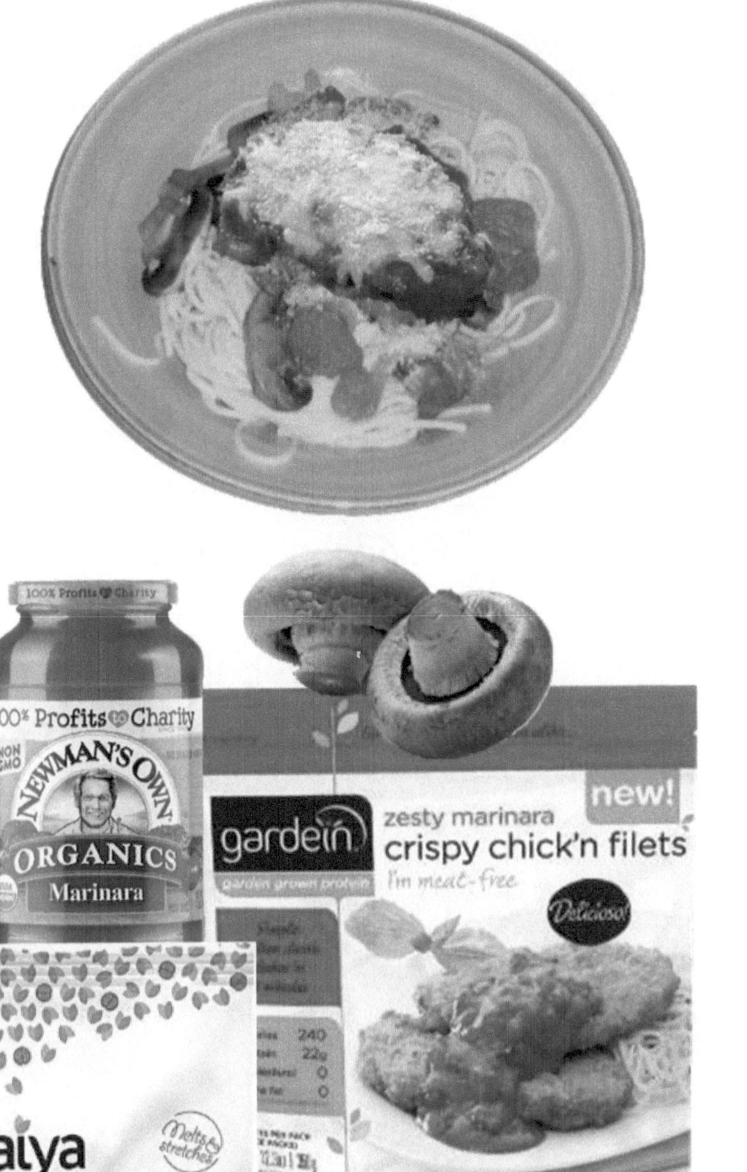

100% Profits to Charity
NON GMO
NEWMAN'S OWN
ORGANICS
Marinara
gardein
garden grown protein
zesty marinara
crispy chick'n filets
I'm meat-free
new!
Delicioso!
240
22g
daiya
deliciously dairy
Dairy, lactose and casein free
Gluten and soy free
Cholesterol free
mozzarel
style shre
0   0   0
Organic
Great Value
USDA ORGANIC
Spaghetti
macaroni product
product of Italy
NET WT 17.6 OZ (1 LB 1.6 OZ) 500g

SWEET POTATOES & GREEN BEANS

1. organic sweet potato baked

2. organic green beans

3. earth balance butter substitute

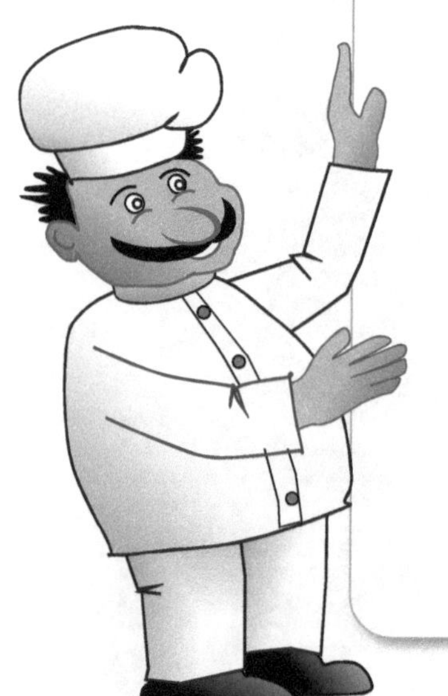

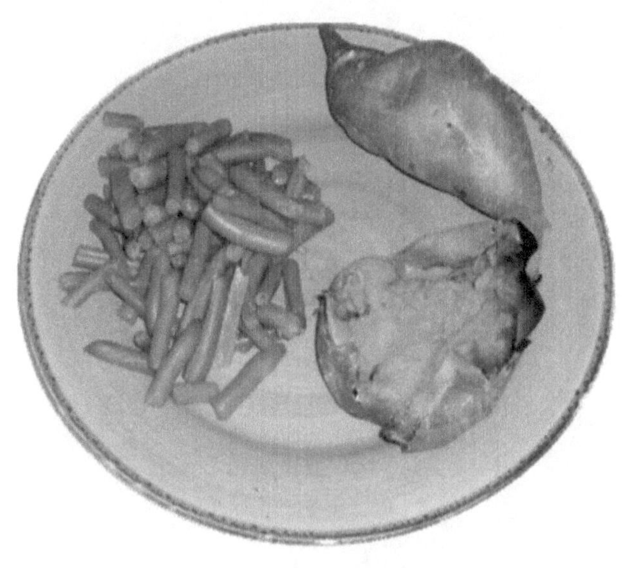

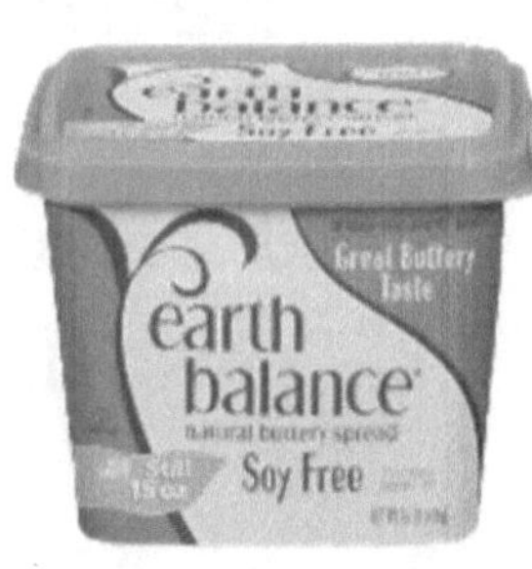
Organic
Great Value
NO SALT ADDED
Cut Green
Beans
USDA
ORGANIC
NET WT 14.5 OZ (411g)

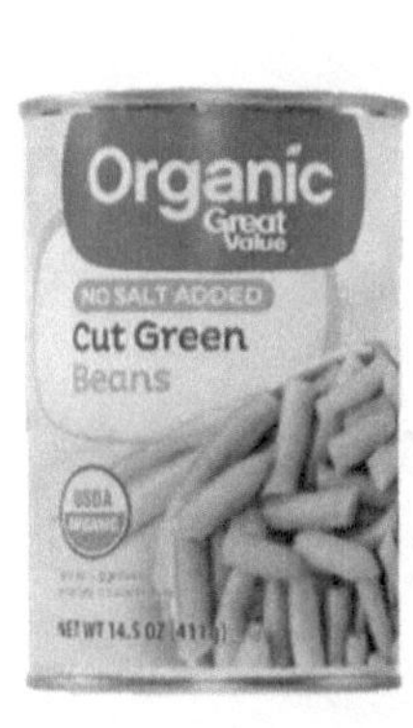
Balance
Soy Free
Great Buttery
Taste
earth
balance
natural buttery spread
Soy Free

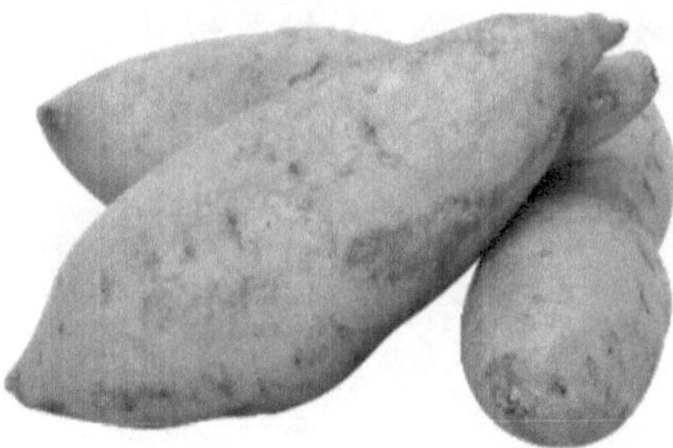

CAULIFLOWER & POTATOES

1. organic Yukon gold potatoes

2. organic cauliflower

3. organic curry powder

4. organic onion

(steam 1-3 or bake)

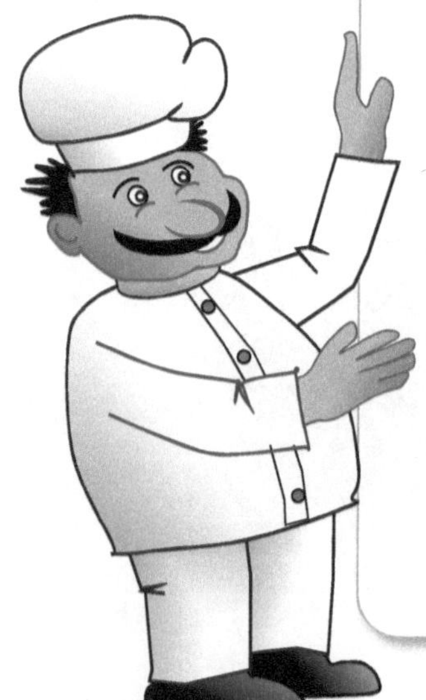

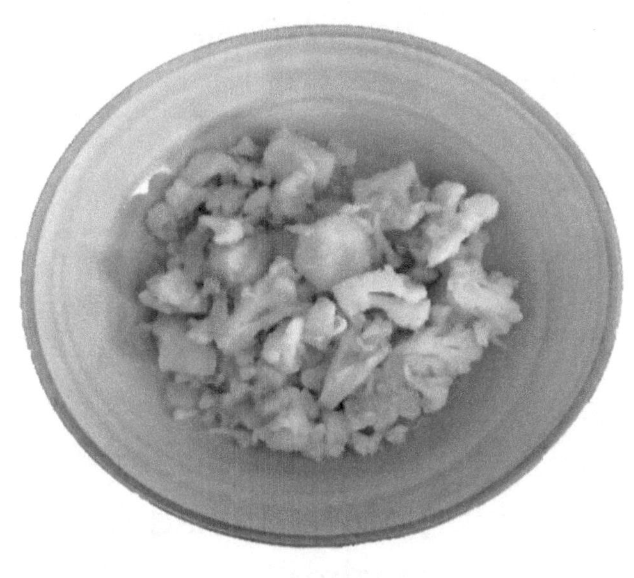

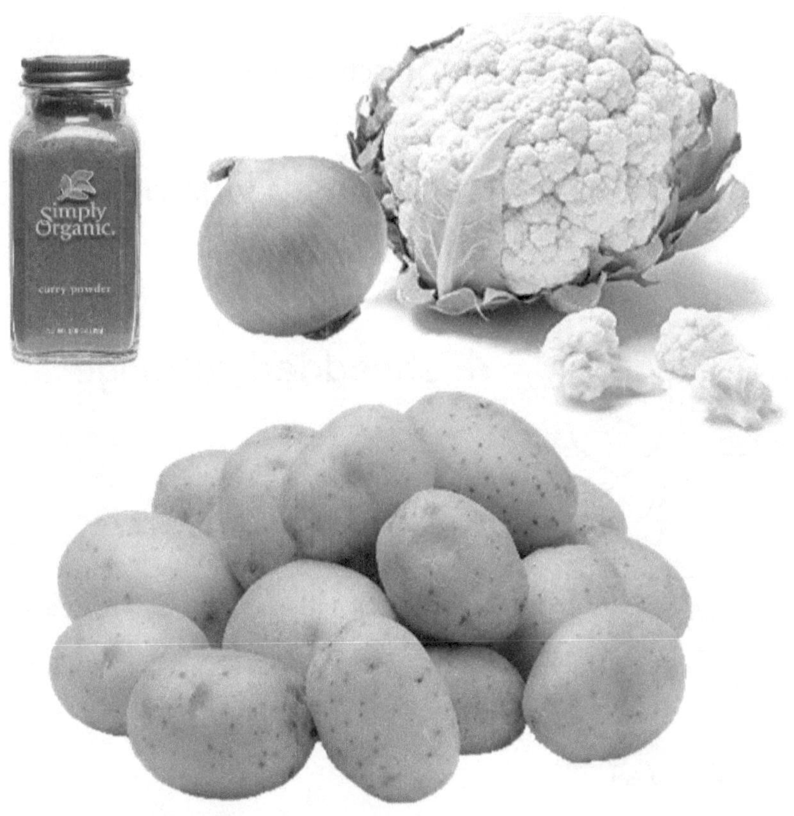

SWEET POTATO & BLACK BEAN TORTILLA

1. organic sweet potato (baked & mashed)

2. organic black beans

3. organic flour or corn tortilla

4. shredded cabbage

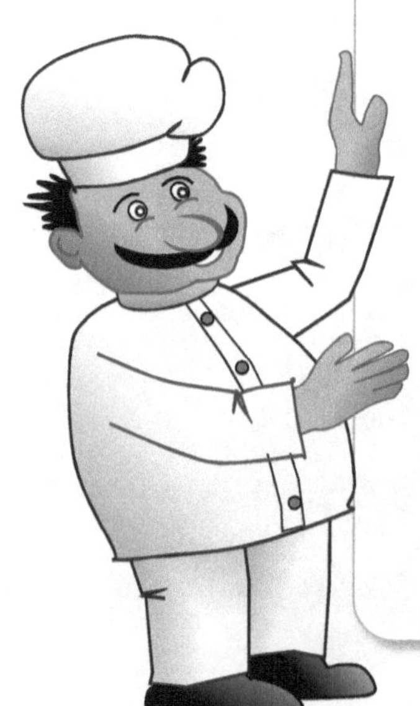

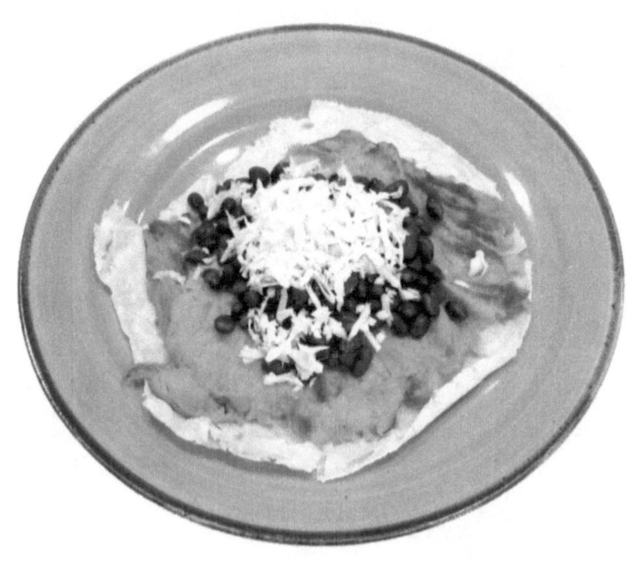

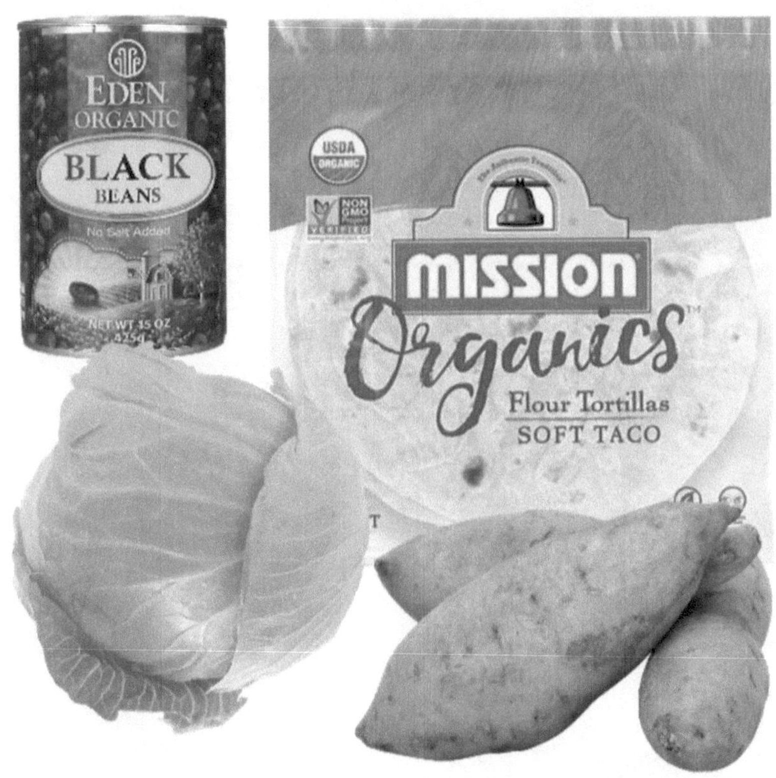
EDEN
ORGANIC
BLACK
BEANS
No Salt Added
NET WT 15 OZ
425g
USDA
ORGANIC
NON
GMO
mission
Organics
Flour Tortillas
SOFT TACO

HUMMUS & BROCCOLI ROLL

1. Naan garlic bread
(regular or gluten-
free)

2. organic red
pepper hummus

3. organic broccoli
steamed, chopped

*(fold it over like a
burrito or wrap)*

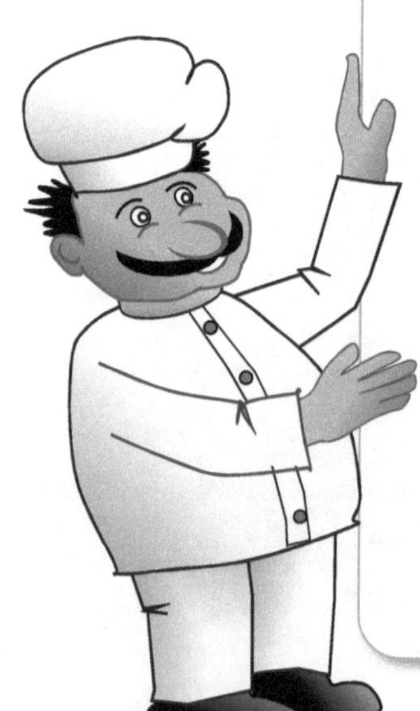

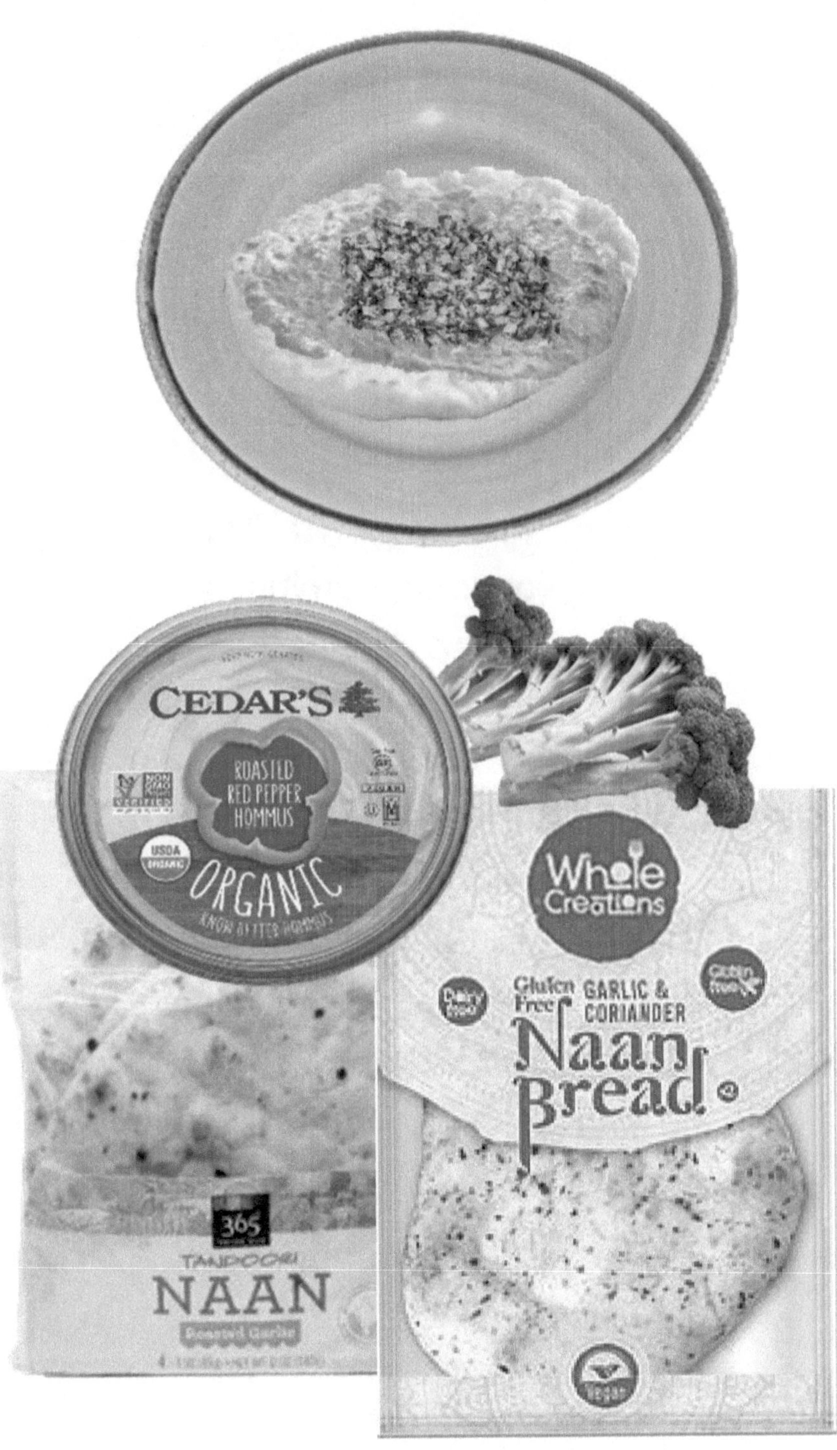
CEDAR'S
ROASTED RED PEPPER HOMMUS
NON GMO
PROJECT VERIFIED
USDA ORGANIC
ORGANIC
Whole Creations
Gluten Free
GARLIC & CORIANDER
Naan Bread
365
TANDOORI
NAAN

ZUCCHINI & PASTA

1. organic spaghetti noodles

2. Newman's Own organic marinara sauce

3. nutritional yeast (grated parmesan cheese substitute)

4. organic zucchini (sliced and sautéed)

ADD BROCCOLI

5. organic broccoli

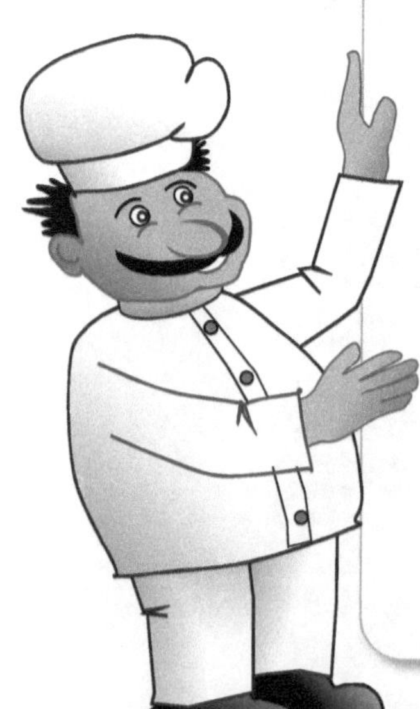

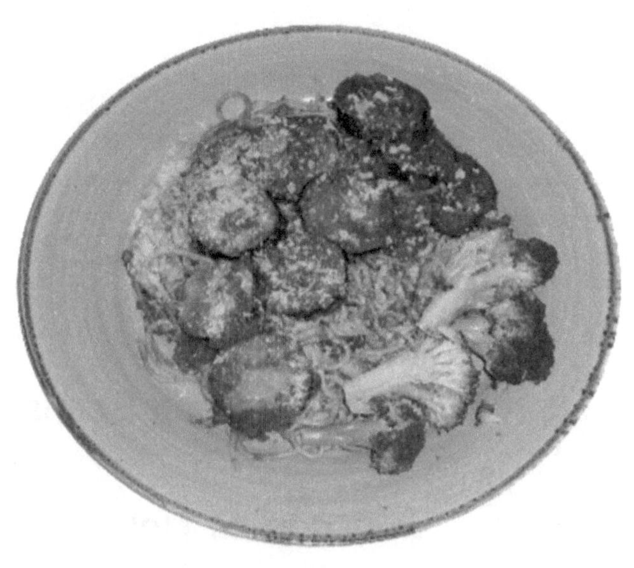

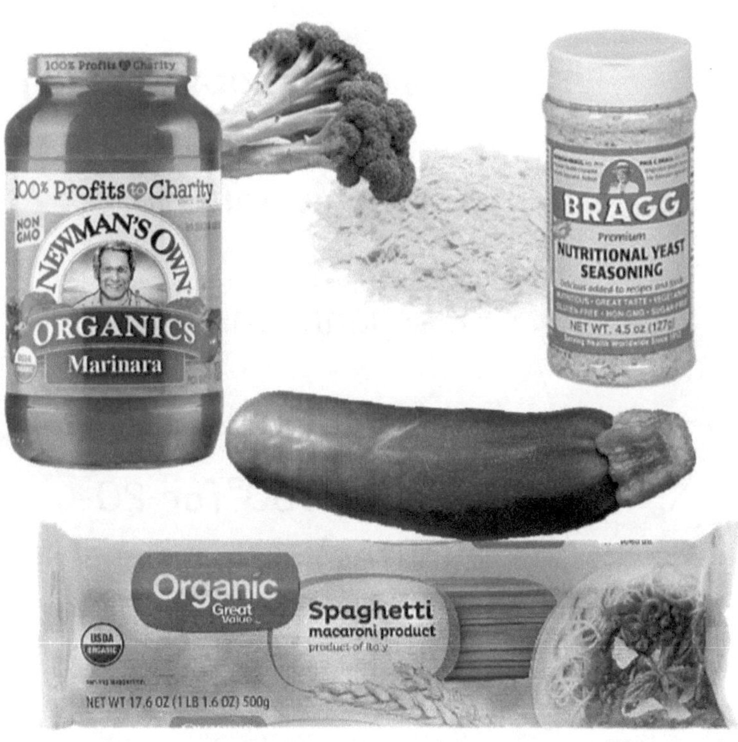
100% Profits Charity
100% Profits Charity
NON GMO
NEWMAN'S OWN
ORGANICS
Marinara
BRAGG
Premium
NUTRITIONAL YEAST
SEASONING
NET WT. 4.5 oz (127g)
USDA ORGANIC
Organic
Great Value
Spaghetti
macaroni product
product of Italy
NET WT 17.6 OZ (1 LB 1.6 OZ) 500g

MEXICAN PIZZA

1. Amy's Organic
Refried Black Beans

2. organics flour
tortilla

3. organic baby spinach

4. organic tomato

5. organic onion

(add toppings then
bake at 360°for 20
minutes)

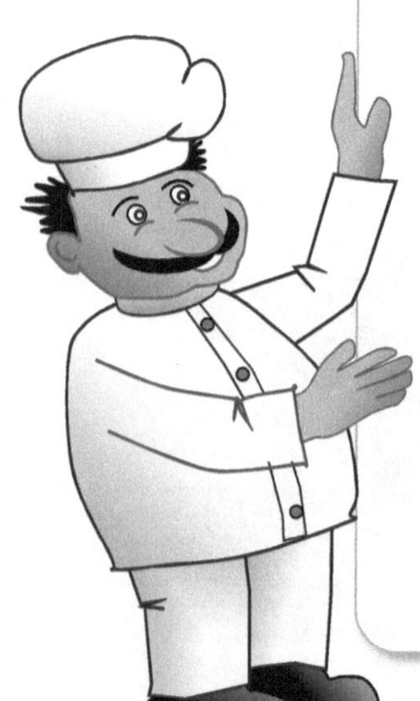

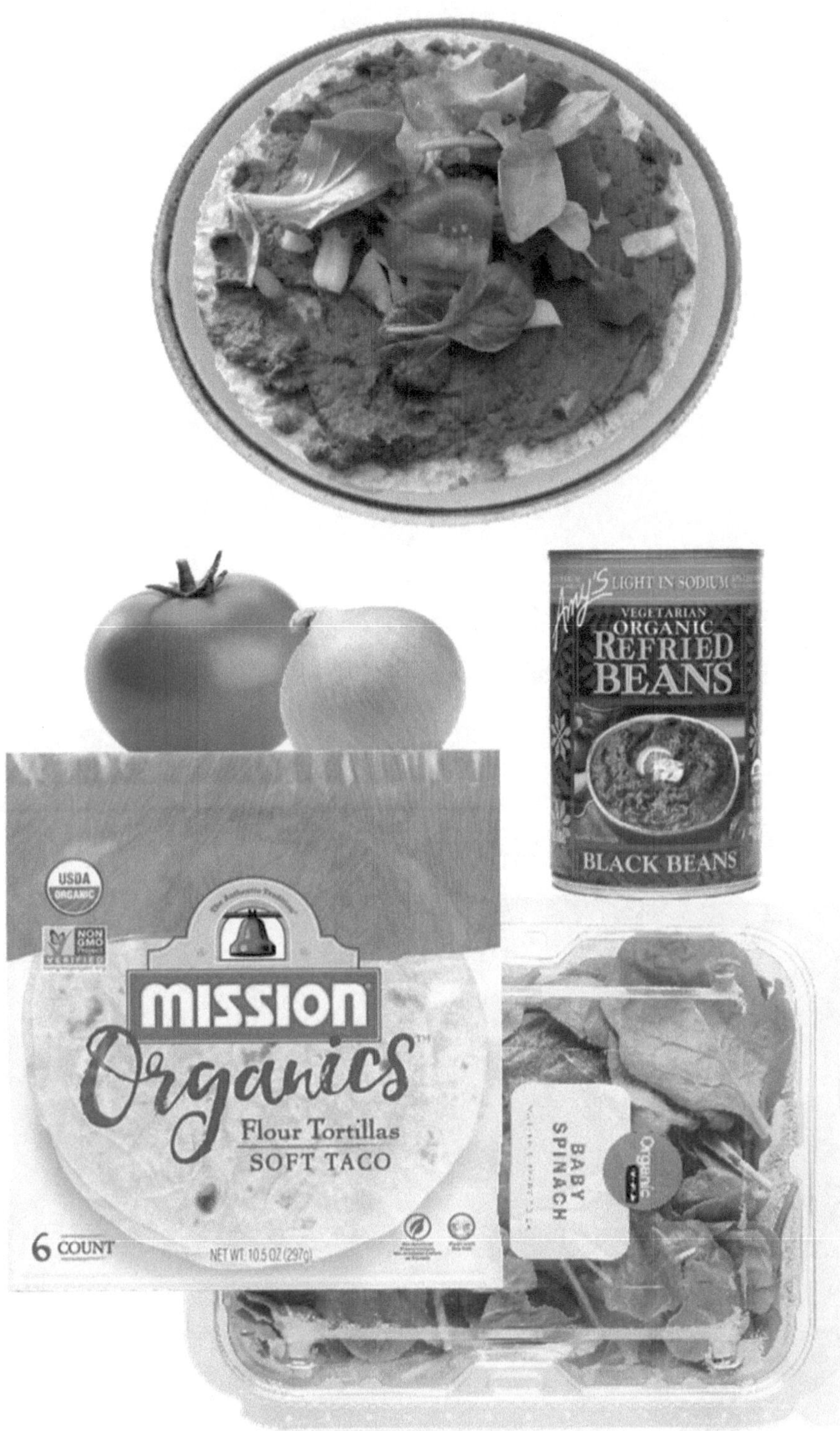
USDA ORGANIC
NON GMO Project VERIFIED
mission
Organics
Flour Tortillas
SOFT TACO
6 COUNT
NET WT. 10.5 OZ (297g)
Amy's LIGHT IN SODIUM
VEGETARIAN
ORGANIC
REFRIED
BEANS
BLACK BEANS
Organic
BABY SPINACH

CHICKEN TENDERS & STEAK FRIES

1. gardein crispy tenders chicken substitute

2. organic steak cut fries

3. Newman's Own Honey Mustard

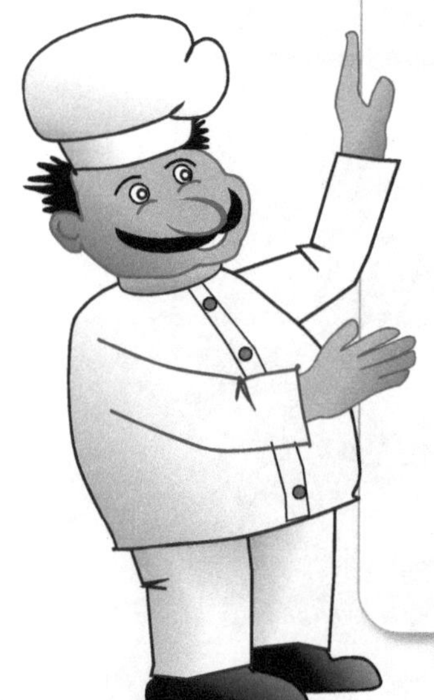

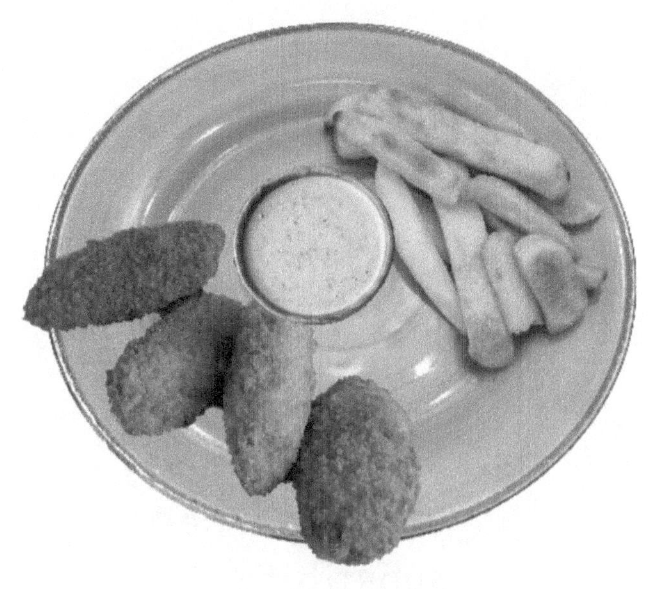

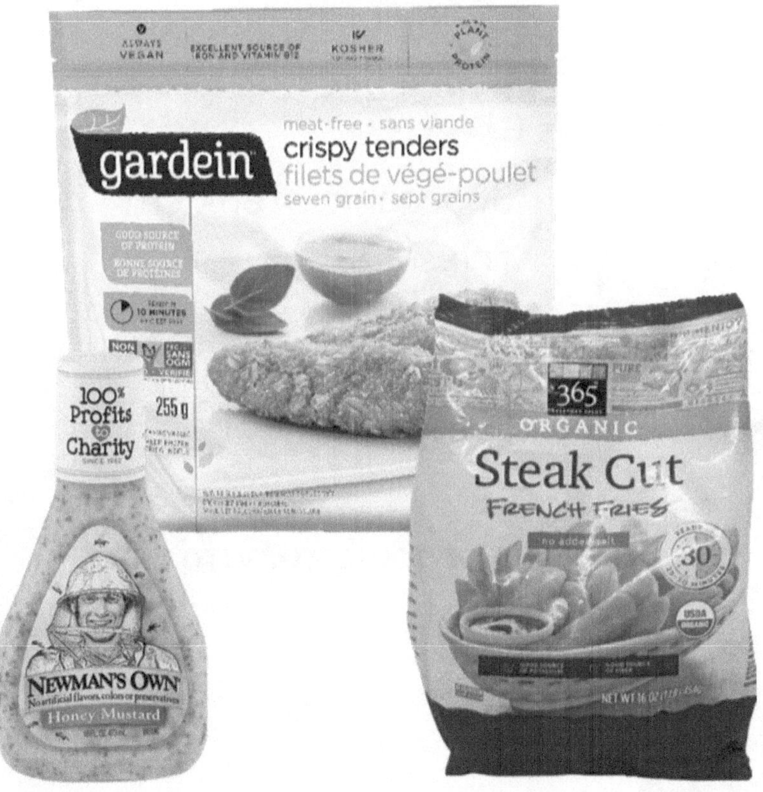
ALWAYS VEGAN
EXCELLENT SOURCE OF IRON AND VITAMIN B12
KOSHER
PLANT PROTEIN
meat-free · sans viande
gardein
crispy tenders
filets de végé-poulet
seven grain · sept grains
GOOD SOURCE OF PROTEIN
BONNE SOURCE DE PROTÉINES
READY IN 10 MINUTES
NON GMO SANS OGM
100% Profits to Charity
255 g
NEWMAN'S OWN
No artificial flavors, colors or preservatives
Honey Mustard
365
ORGANIC
Steak Cut
FRENCH FRIES
no added salt
READY IN 30
USDA ORGANIC
NET WT 16 OZ

CHICKEN SANDWICH & STEAK FRIES

1. gardein crispy chick'n patties substitute

2. organic bun

3. organic steak cut fries

4. organic Romaine lettuce

5.organic tomato

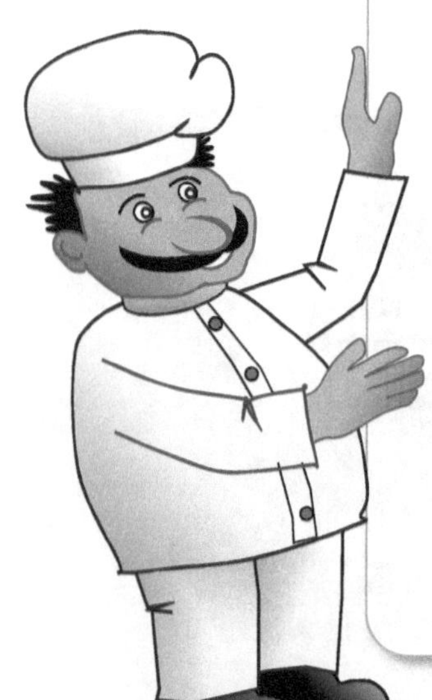

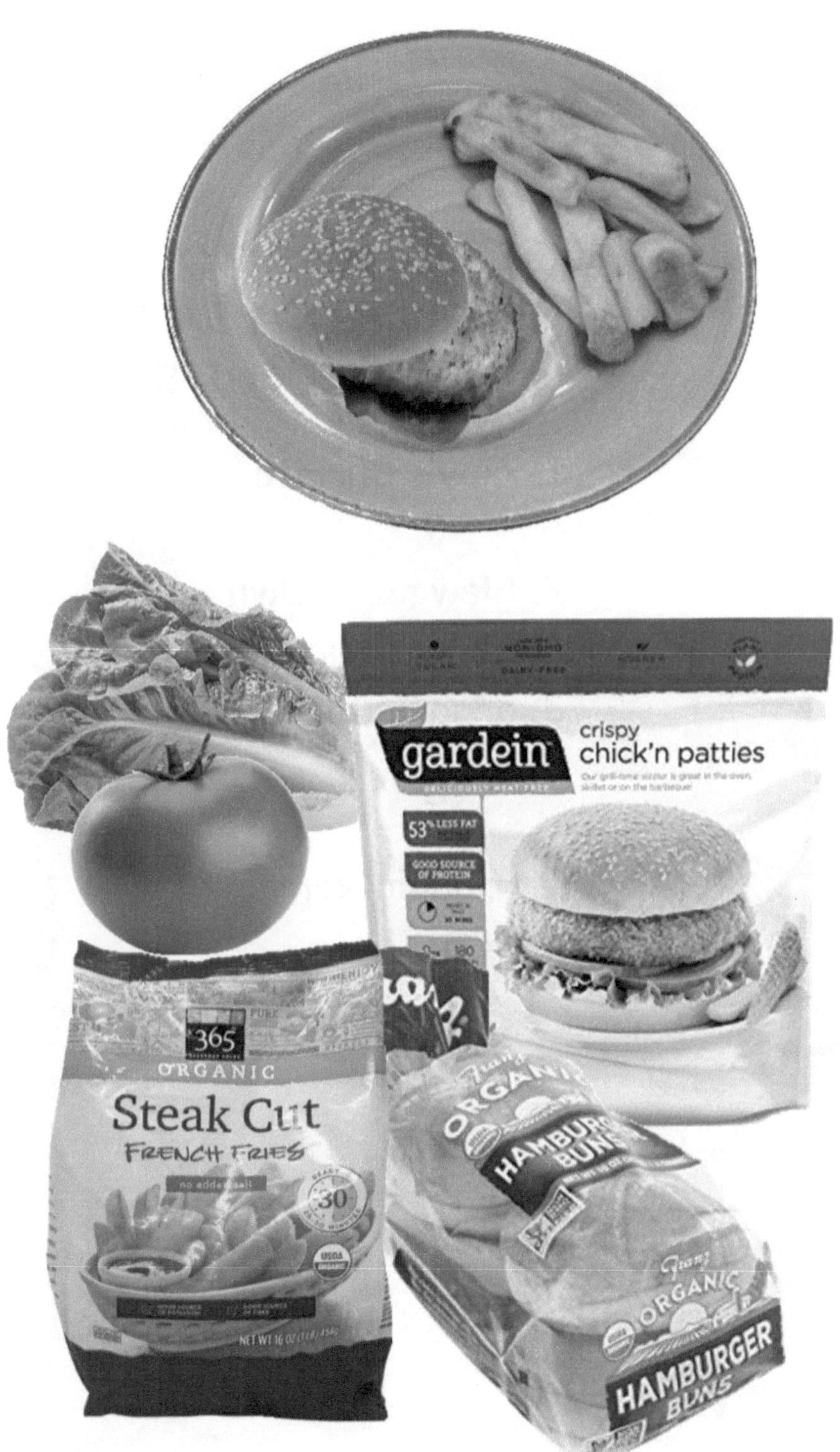

gardein
crispy
chick'n patties
53% LESS FAT
GOOD SOURCE
OF PROTEIN
365
ORGANIC
Steak Cut
FRENCH FRIES
no added salt
30
NET WT 16 OZ
ORGANIC
HAMBURGER BUNS
ORGANIC
HAMBURGER
BUNS

BEAN BURRITO, LETTUCE, SALSA & TORTILLA CHIPS

1. Amy's Burrito

2. Newman's Own
Medium Chunky Salsa
3. organic blue corn
Chips

4. organic Romaine
lettuce

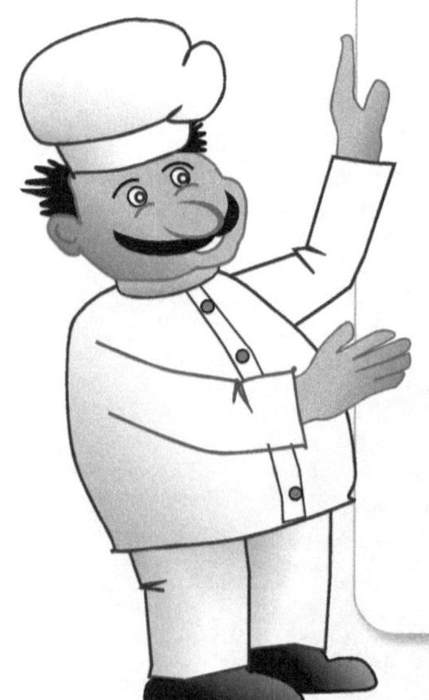

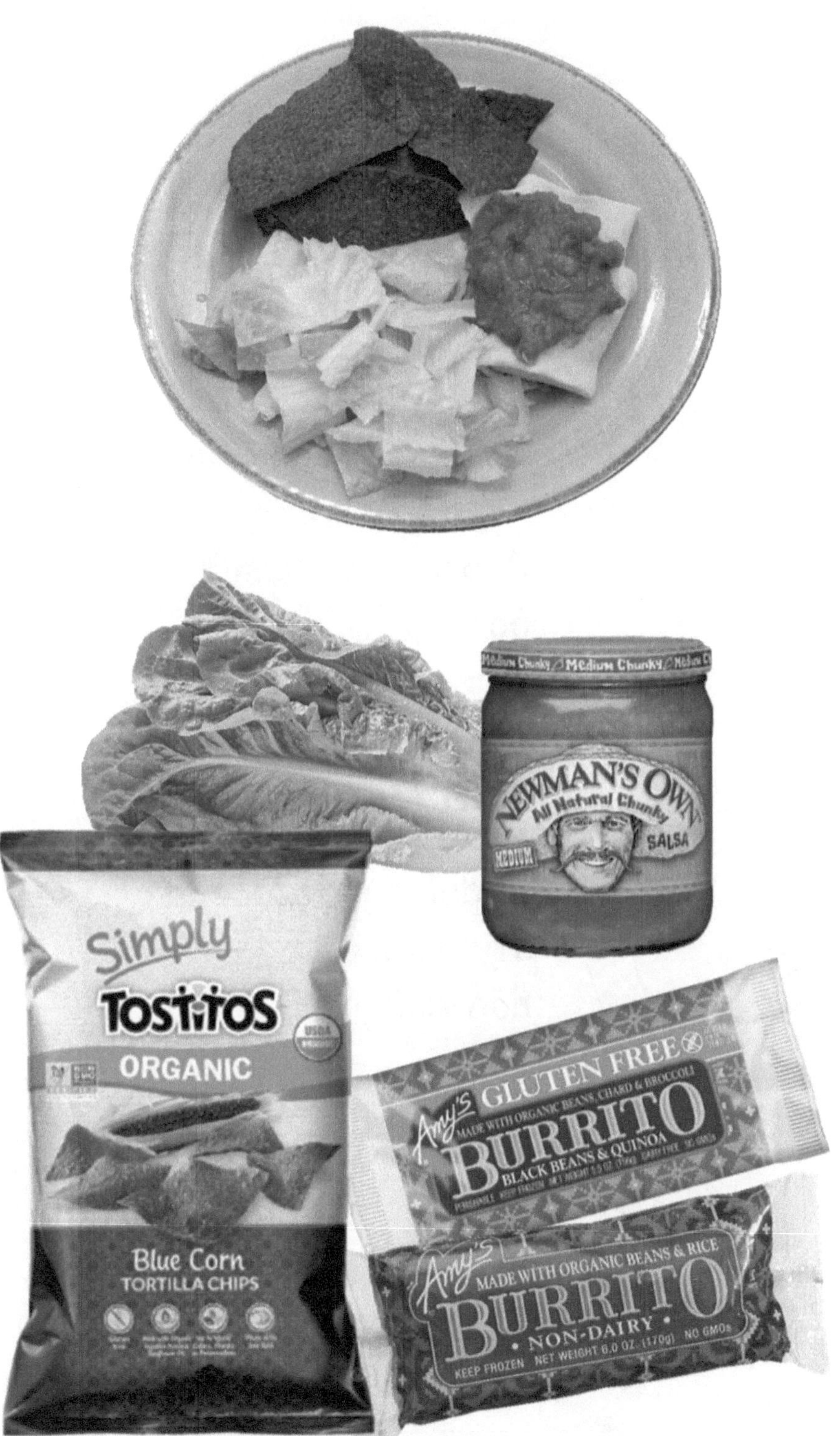

Simply
Tostitos
ORGANIC
Blue Corn
TORTILLA CHIPS
NEWMAN'S OWN
All Natural Chunky
MEDIUM
SALSA
Medium Chunky
Amy's
GLUTEN FREE
MADE WITH ORGANIC BEANS, CHARD & BROCCOLI
BURRITO
BLACK BEANS & QUINOA
Amy's
MADE WITH ORGANIC BEANS & RICE
BURRITO
NON-DAIRY
KEEP FROZEN   NET WEIGHT 6.0 OZ. (170g)   NO GMOs

BAKED POTATO & CHILLI

1. Amy's Organic Chili or Black Bean Chili

2. organic Russet potato

ADD MOZZARELLA

3. daiya mozzarella style shreds non-dairy

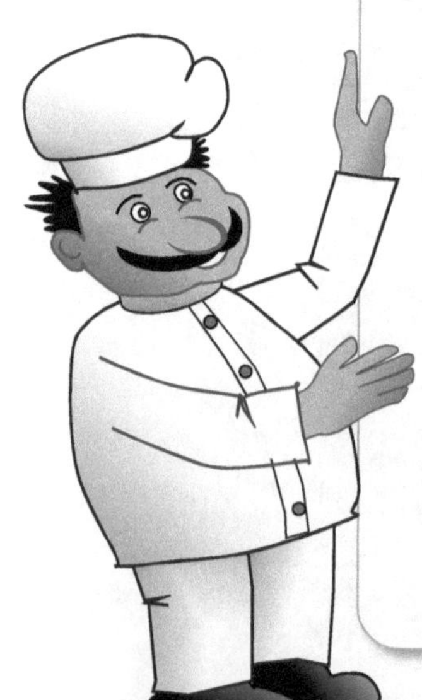

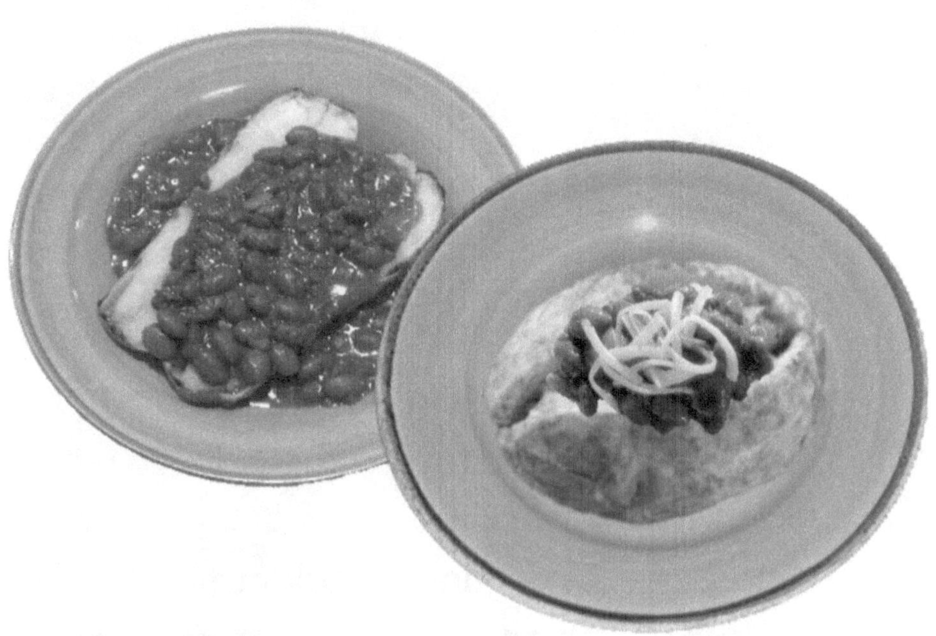

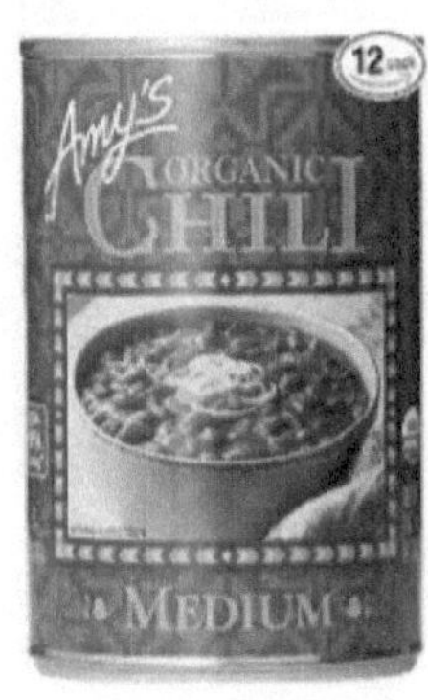
Amy's
ORGANIC
CHILI
MEDIUM

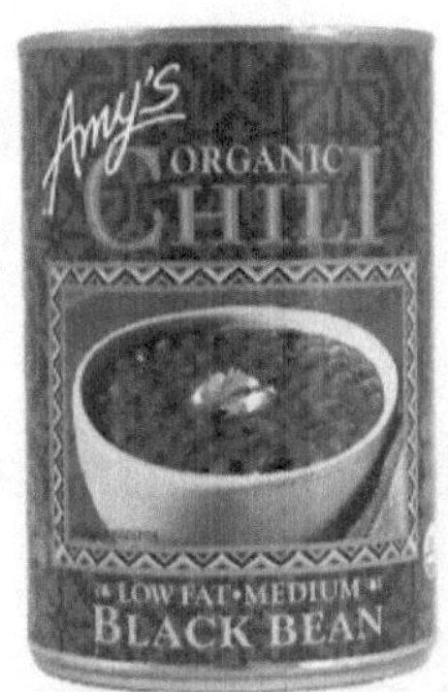
Amy's
ORGANIC
CHILI
LOW FAT · MEDIUM
BLACK BEAN

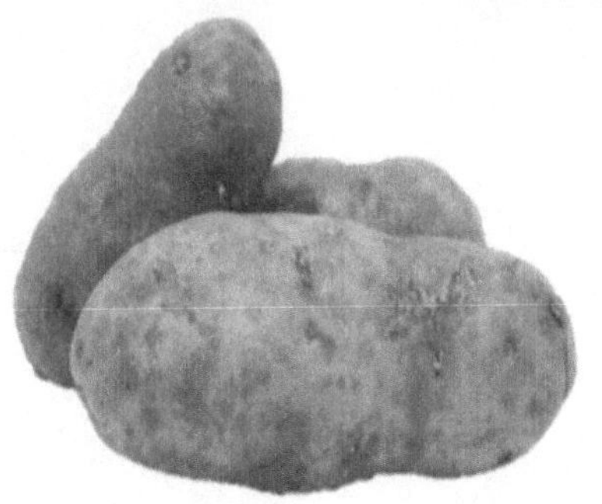

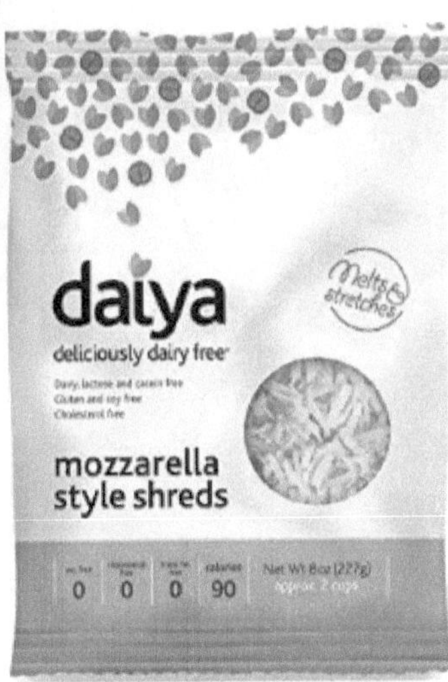
daiya
deliciously dairy free
mozzarella
style shreds
Net Wt 8oz (227g)

BURGER & STEAK FRIES

1. gardein burger substitute

2. organic steak cut fries

3. organic tomato or ketchup or mustard

4. oranic burger bun

5. organic Romaine lettuce

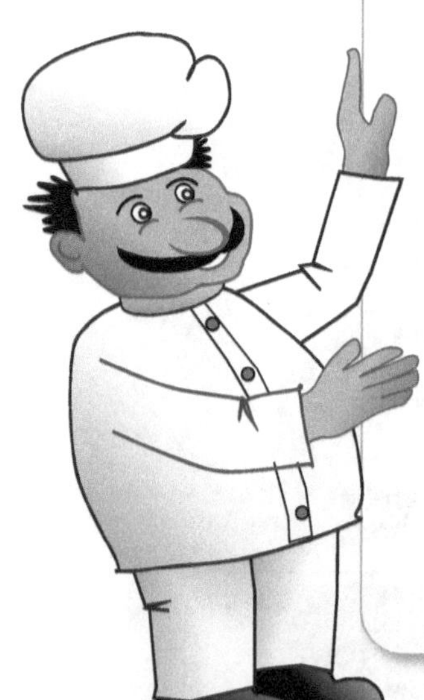

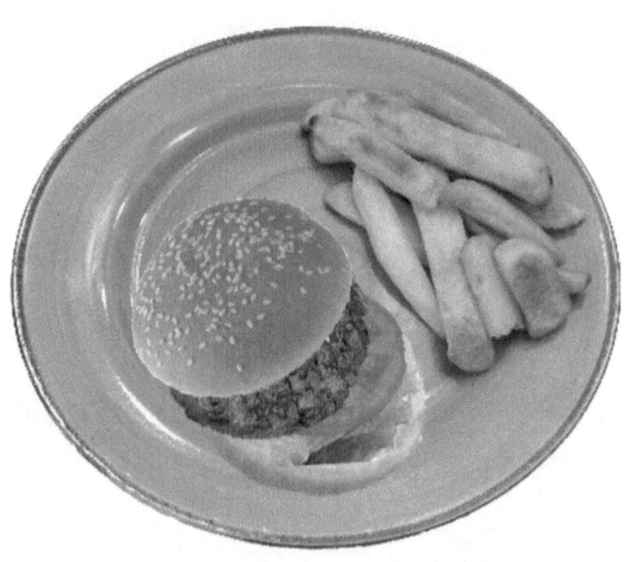
365
ORGANIC
Steak Cut
FRENCH FRIES
no added salt
30
USDA ORGANIC
NET WT 16 OZ (1 LB) 454g
ORGANIC
HAMBURGER BUNS
ORGANIC
HAMBURGER
BUNS
For meat and veggie lovers alike
new!
gardein
the ultimate
beefless burger
I'm meat-free
65% less fat
130
17g
0
0

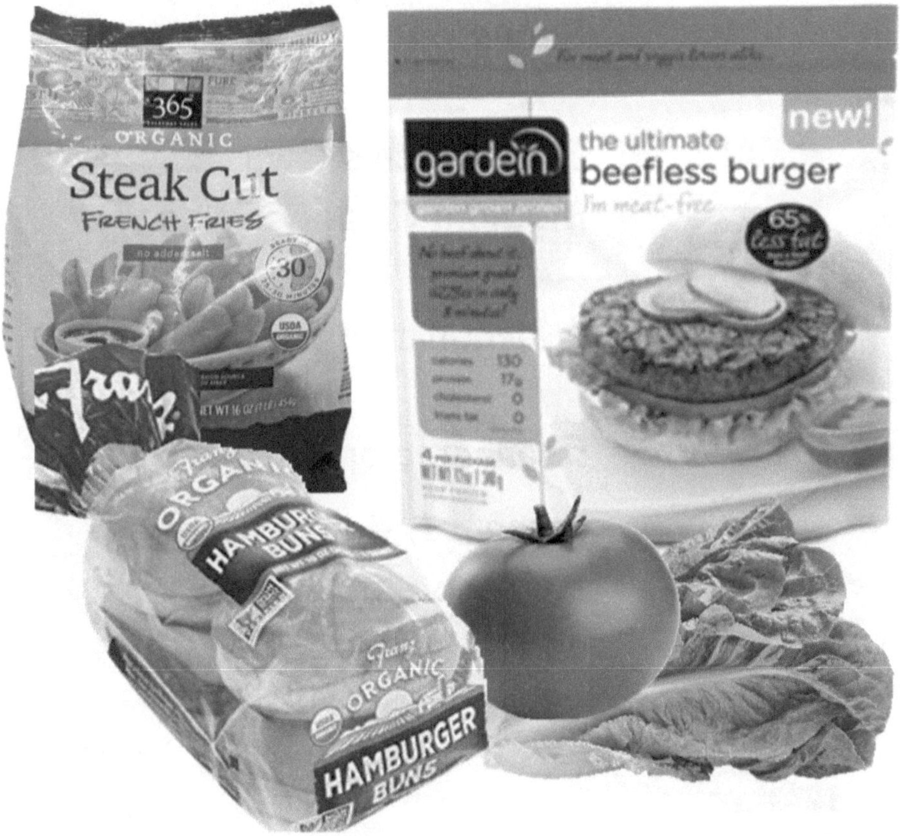

POTATO-SALSA SOUP

1. organic Yukon gold potatoes

2. Eden Organic Navy Beans

3. Newman's Own Medium Chunky Salsa

4. organic tomato

5. organic onion

(steam 1, 4 & 5, when softened, add 2 & 3 and stir)

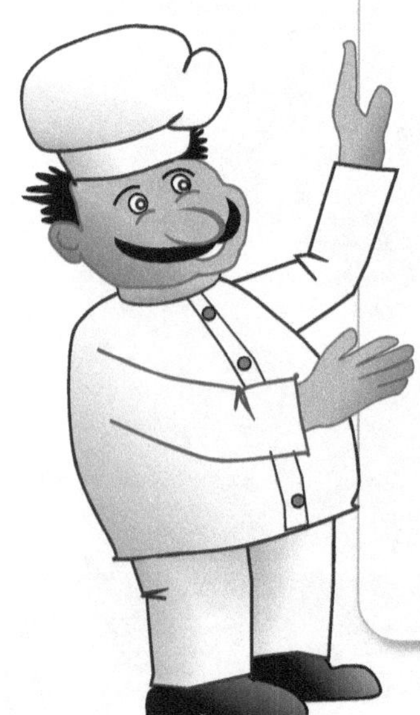

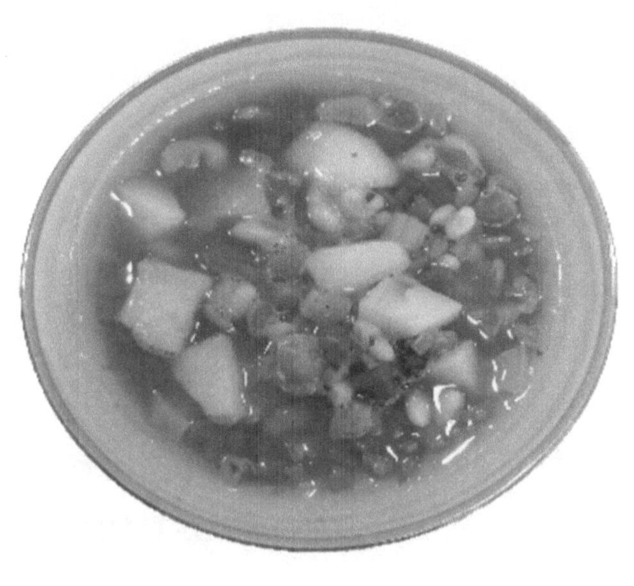

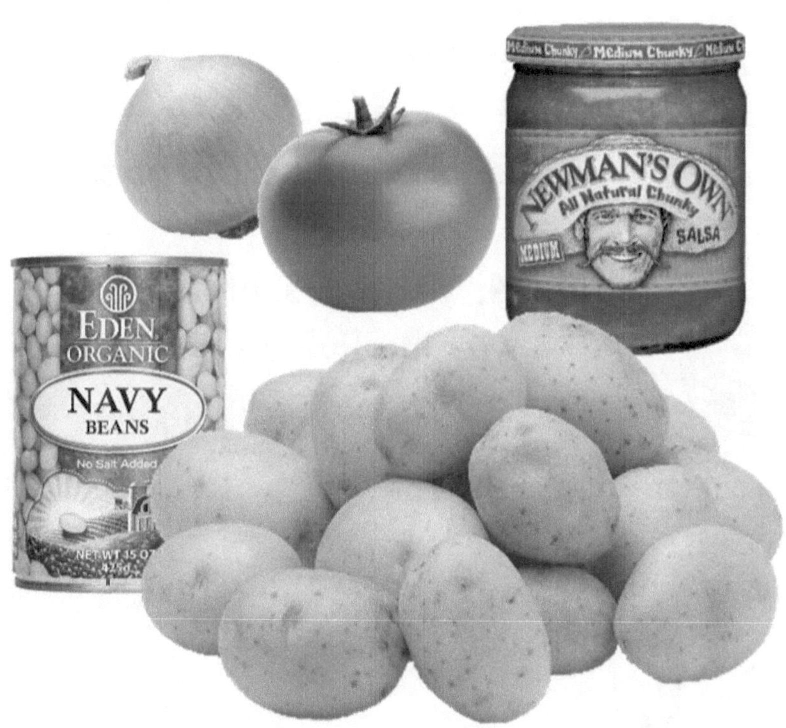

SAUSAGE, POTATOES & BELL PEPPERS

1. Gimme Lean ground sausage substitute

2. organic Yukon gold potatoes

3. organic bell pepper

4. Venta Baron extra virgin olive oil or sesame oil for frying sausage

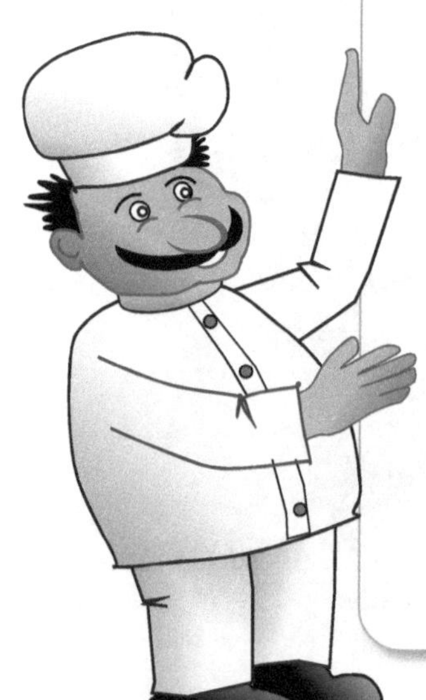

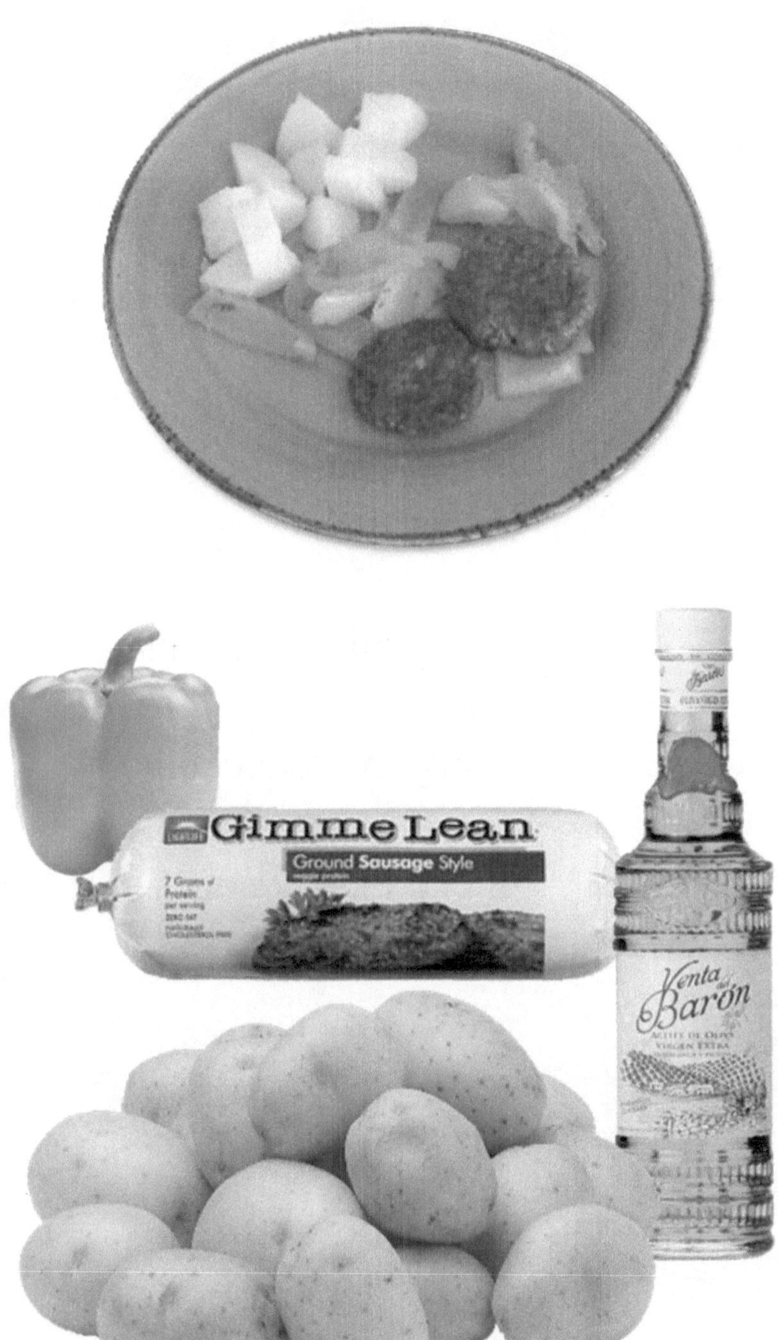

Gimme Lean
Ground Sausage Style
Venta del Barón

CHICKEN, RICE AND BROCCOLI

1. gardein crispy chick'n patties substitute

2. organic brown rice

3. organic broccoli

4. oranic soy sauce

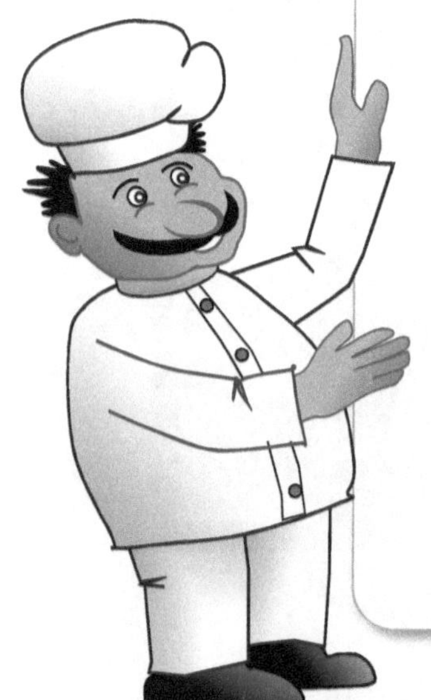

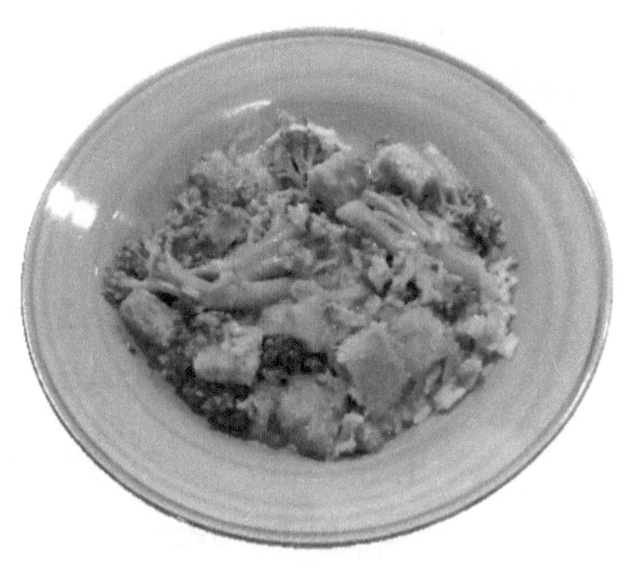

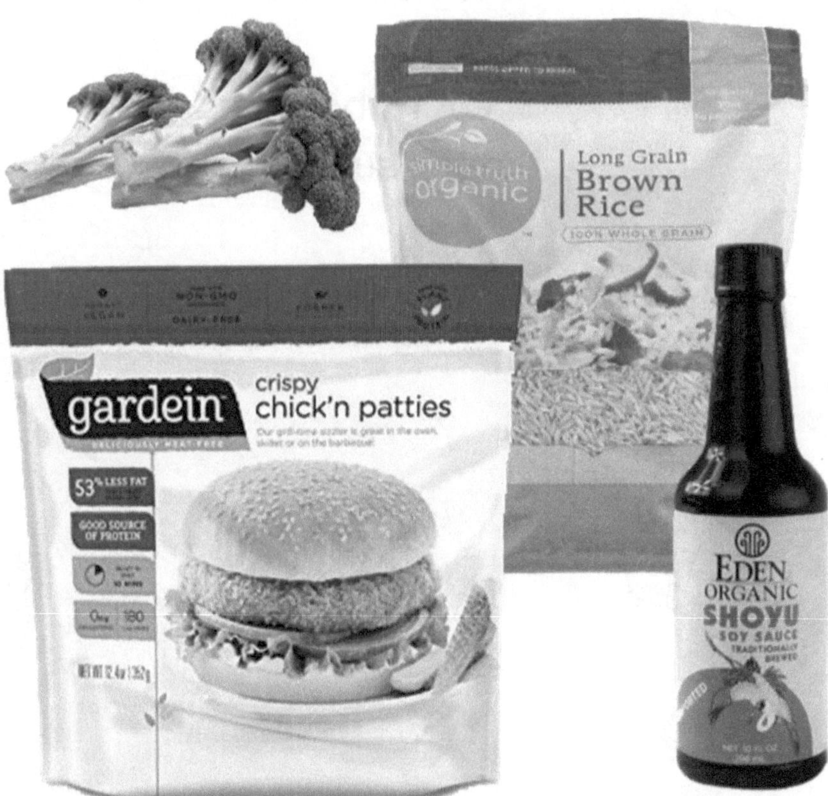

simple truth organic
Long Grain
Brown
Rice
100% WHOLE GRAIN
gardein
crispy
chick'n patties
DELICIOUSLY MEAT-FREE
53% LESS FAT
GOOD SOURCE
OF PROTEIN
EDEN
ORGANIC
SHOYU
SOY SAUCE
TRADITIONALLY
BREWED

STEAMED POTATOES & SWEET PEAS

1. organic
red potatoes

2. organic sweet peas

3. earth balance
butter substitute

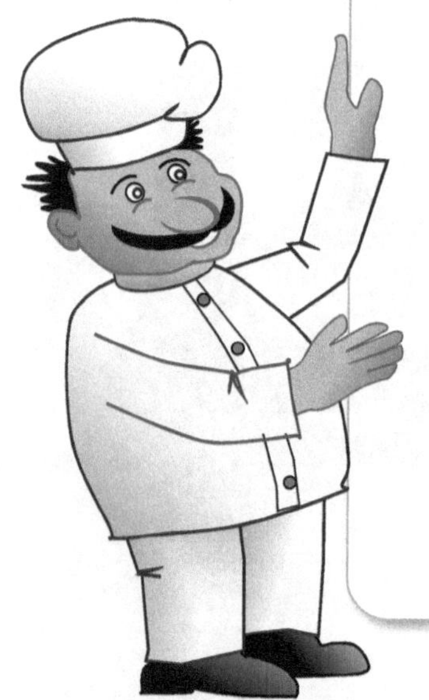

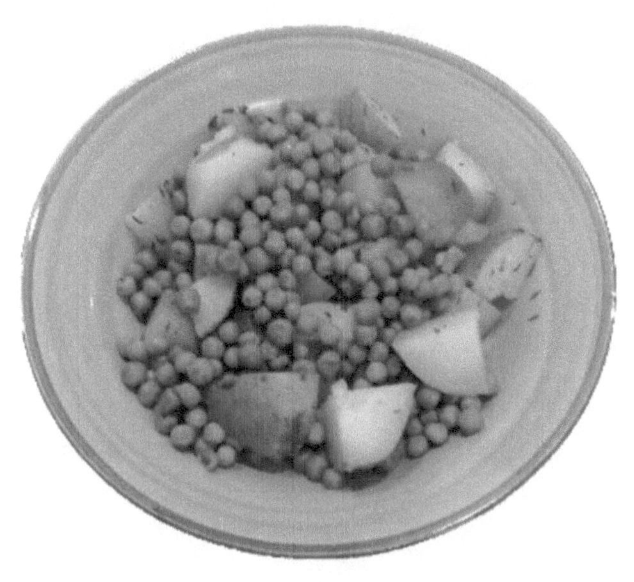

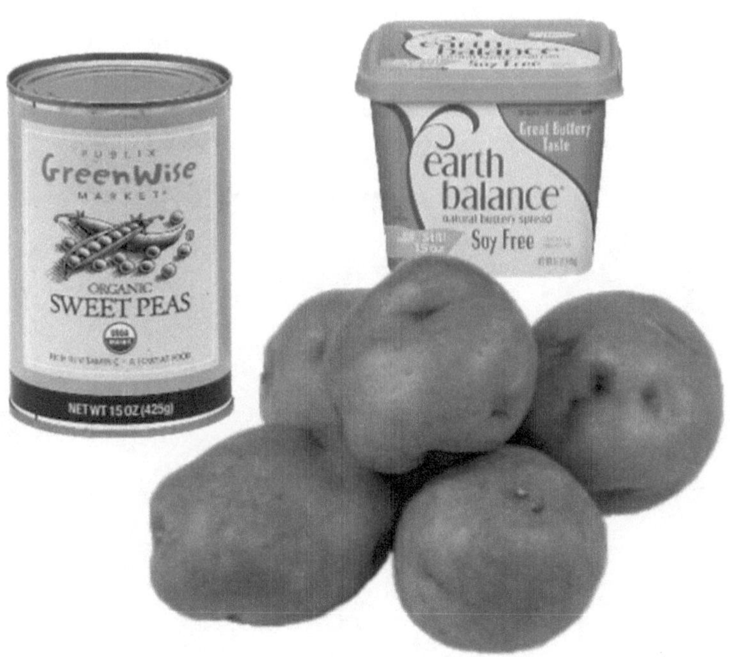
PUBLIX
GreenWise
MARKET
ORGANIC
SWEET PEAS
NET WT 15 OZ (425g)
earth
balance
natural buttery spread
Soy Free
Great Buttery
Taste

THAI RED CURRY

1. Amy's Thai Red Curry

THAI PAD THAI

1. Amy's Thai Pad Thai

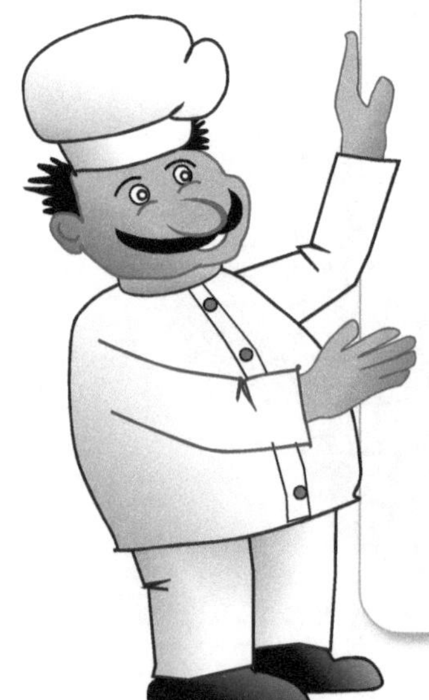

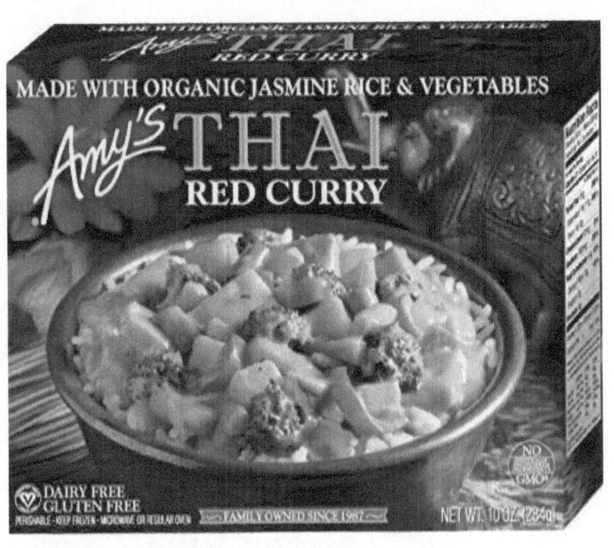
MADE WITH ORGANIC JASMINE RICE & VEGETABLES
Amy's THAI
RED CURRY
DAIRY FREE
GLUTEN FREE
FAMILY OWNED SINCE 1987
NET WT. 10 OZ. (284g)

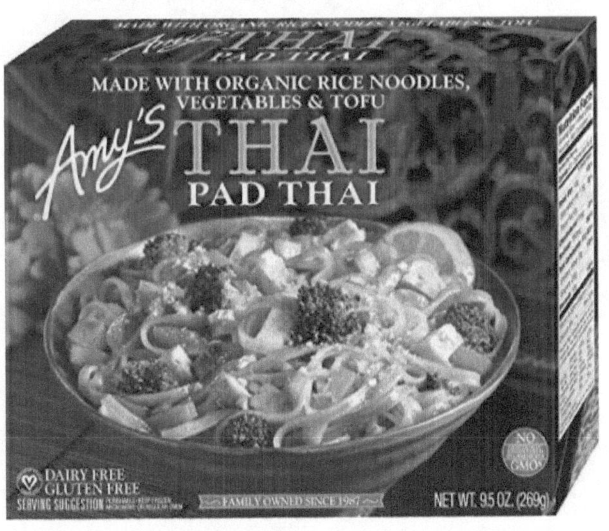
MADE WITH ORGANIC RICE NOODLES,
VEGETABLES & TOFU
Amy's THAI
PAD THAI
DAIRY FREE
GLUTEN FREE
SERVING SUGGESTION
FAMILY OWNED SINCE 1987
NET WT. 9.5 OZ. (269g)

CHILI RELLENO & TORTILLA CHIPS

1. Amy's Casserole Chile Relleno

2. organic Simply Tostitos Blue Corn Tortilla Chips

(Try dipping the chips!)

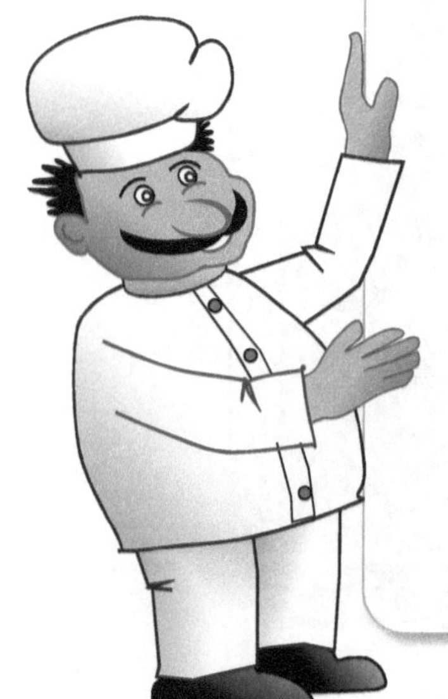

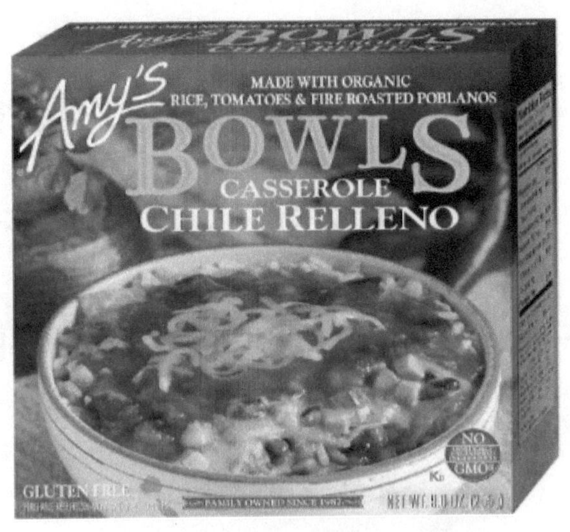

Amy's
MADE WITH ORGANIC
RICE, TOMATOES & FIRE ROASTED POBLANOS
BOWLS
CASSEROLE
CHILE RELLENO
GLUTEN FREE
NO GMO
NET WT. 9.0 OZ (255 g)
FAMILY OWNED SINCE 1987

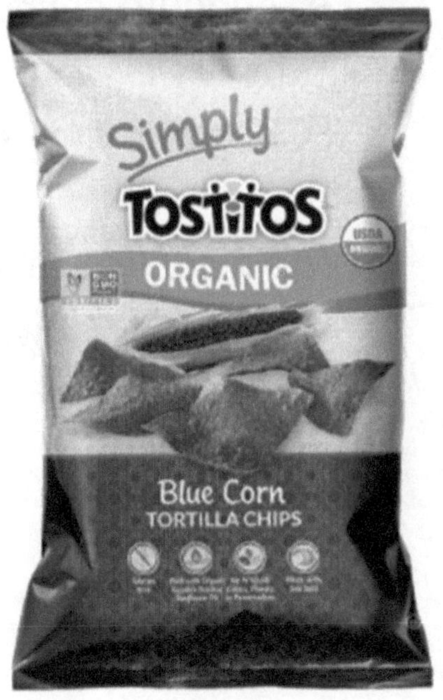

Simply
Tostitos
ORGANIC
Blue Corn
TORTILLA CHIPS

STIR FRIED RICE

1. organic brown rice

2. organic sweet peas

3. organic onion

4. organic carrot

5. organic soy sauce

(add garlic, cayenne, and ginger powder if you want)

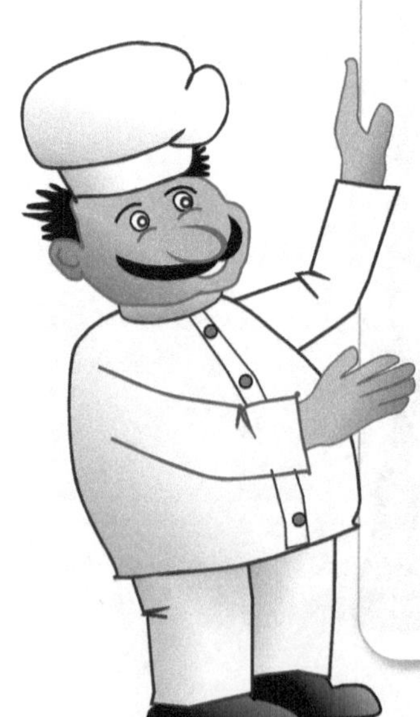

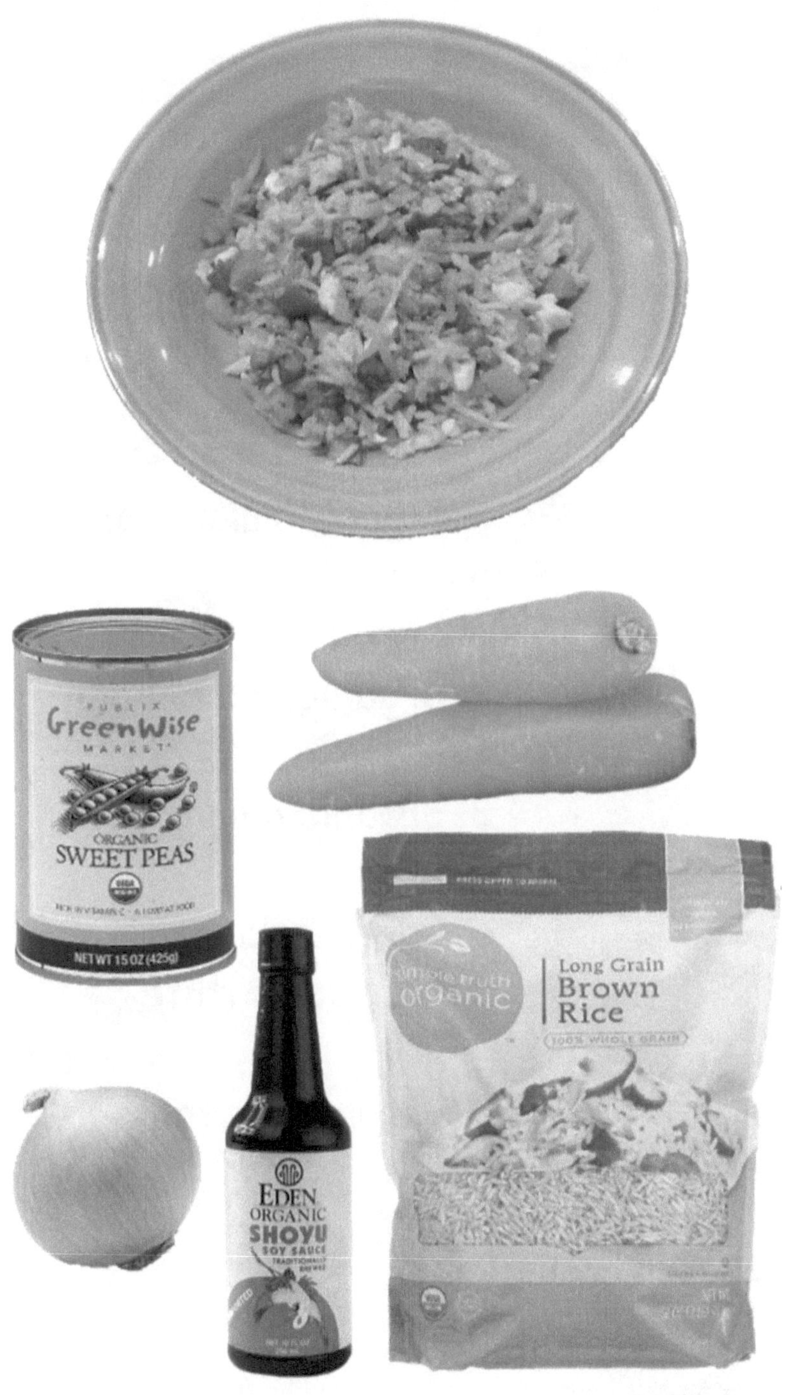

STEAMED POTATOS, GREEN BEANS, ONION & PEPPERS

1. organic Yukon gold potatoes

2. organic red pepper

3. organic onion

4. earth balance butter substitute

5. organic green beans

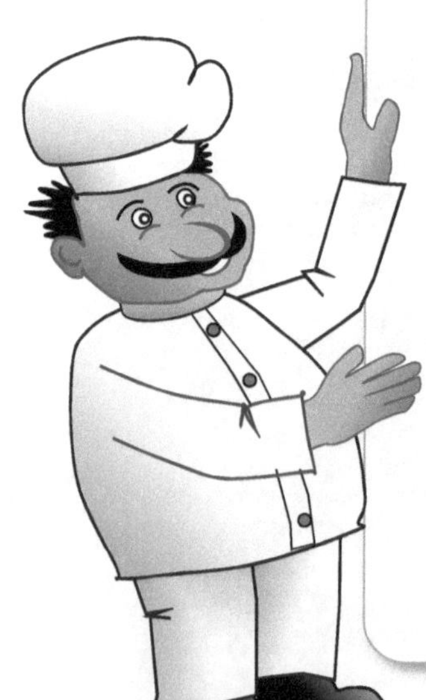

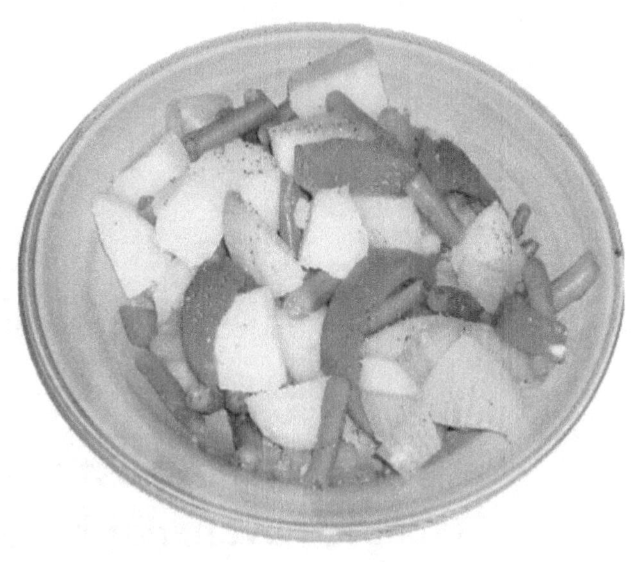

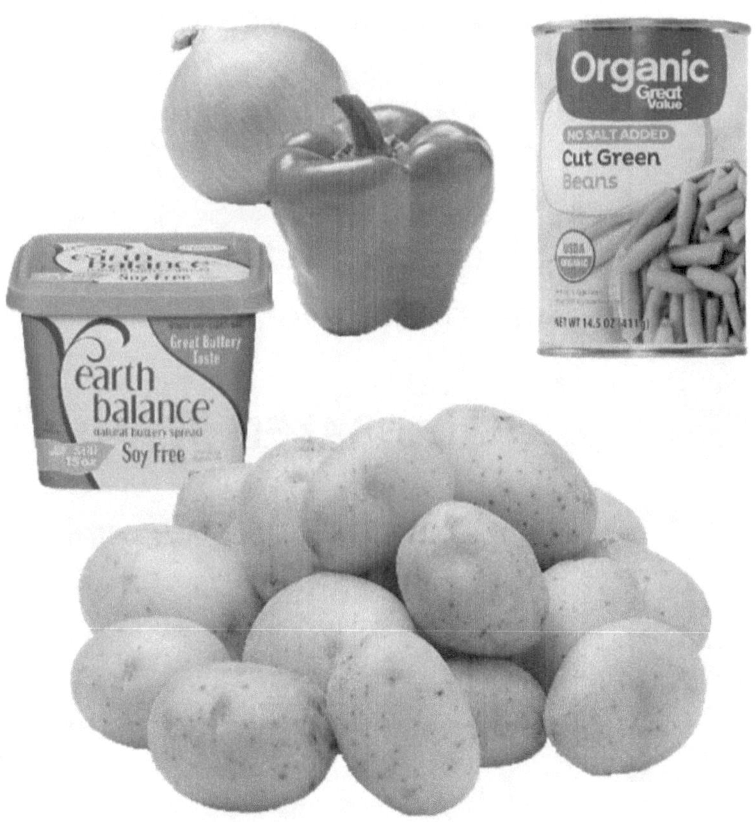

HOTDOG, STEAK FRIES & BAKED BEANS

1. Field Roast Frankfurters substitute (toaster oven, <u>not</u> boiled)

2. organic steak cut fries

3. organic hotdog bun

4. organic ketchup or mustard or onion

ADD BAKED BEANS

5. Walnut Acres Organic Baked Beans

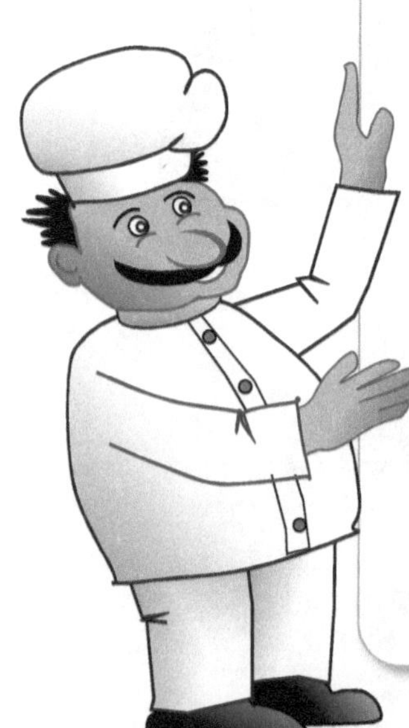

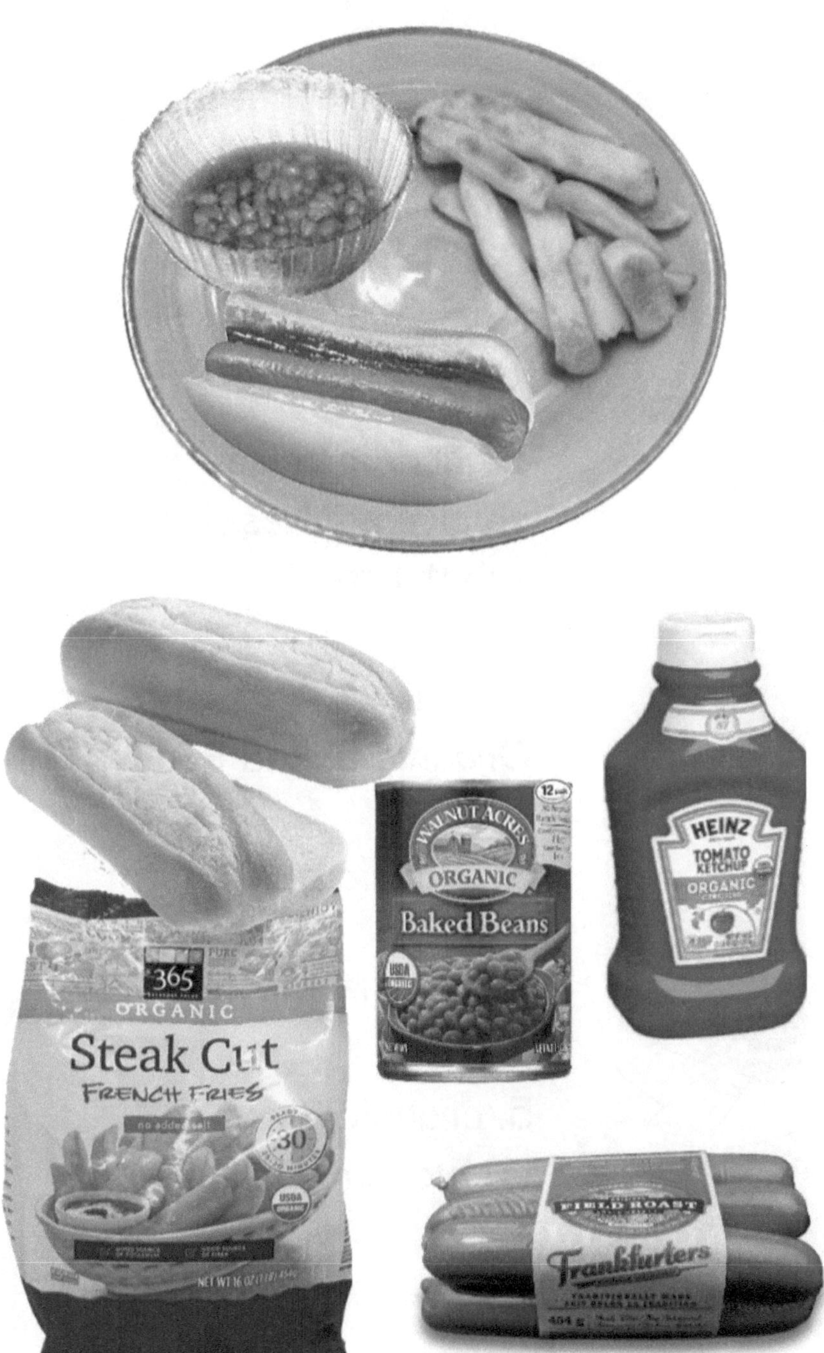

ORGANIC
Baked Beans
HEINZ
TOMATO
KETCHUP
ORGANIC
365
ORGANIC
Steak Cut
FRENCH FRIES
NET WT 16 OZ
FIELD ROAST
Frankfurters
454 g

CHICKEN SANDWICH & BAKED BEANS

1. gardein crispy chick'n patties substitute

2. Walnut Acres Organic Baked Beans

3. organic bun

4. organic tomato

5. organic Romaine lettuce or cucumber

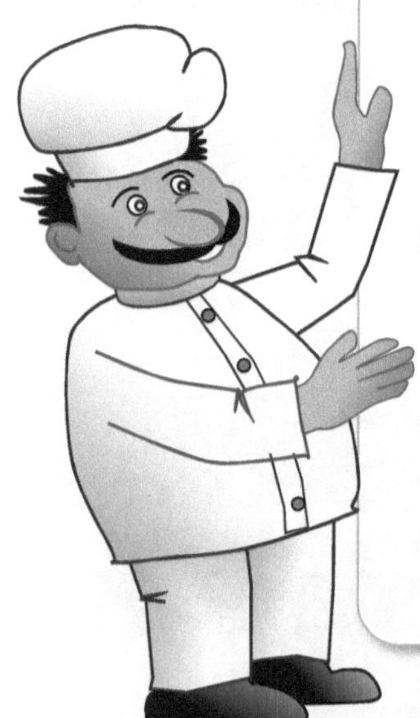

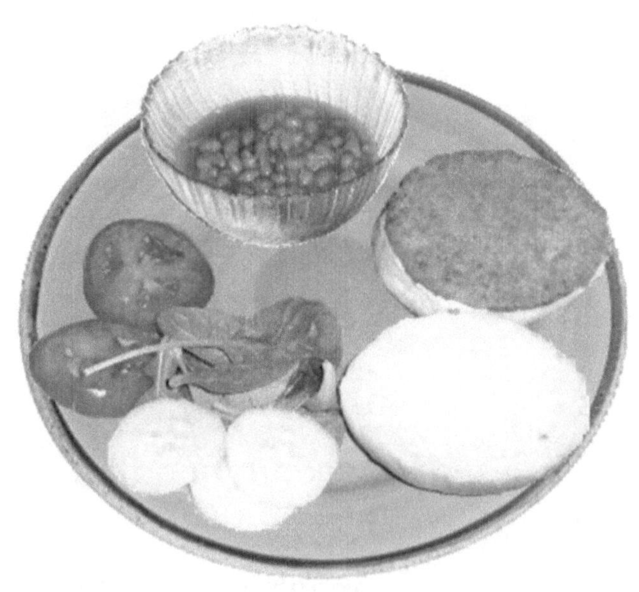

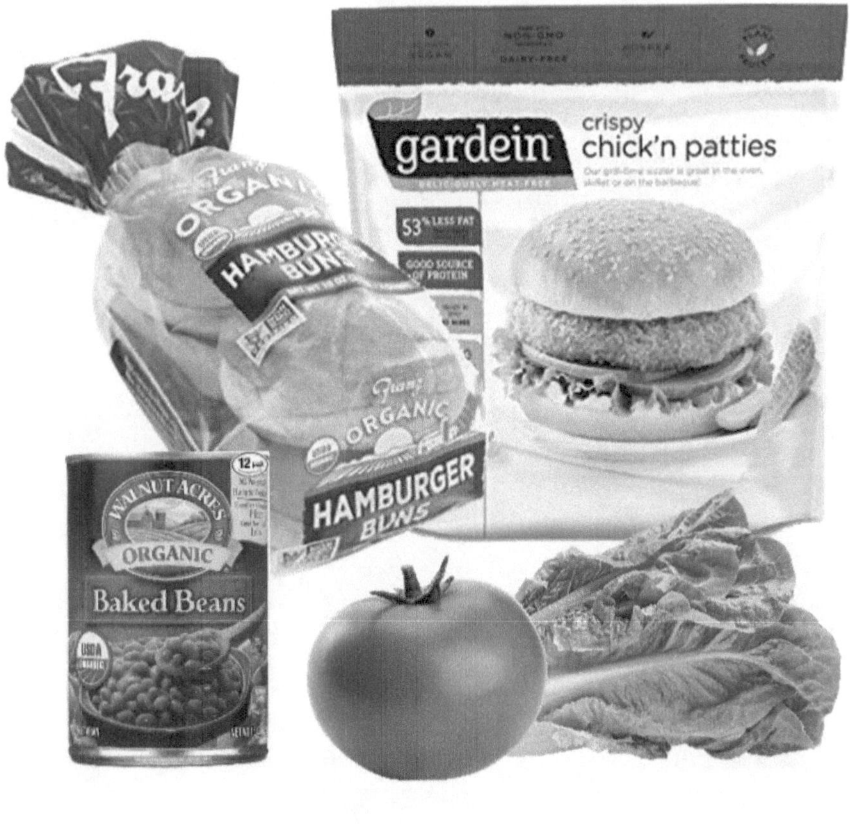

gardein
crispy
chick'n patties
53% LESS FAT
GOOD SOURCE
OF PROTEIN
ORGANIC
HAMBURGER BUNS
ORGANIC
HAMBURGER
BUNS
WALNUT ACRES
ORGANIC
Baked Beans

NOODLES, PEAS, CAULIFLOWER & ONION

1. organic noodles

2. organic sweet peas

3. sautéed organic onion

4.organic cauliflower

5. Venta Baron extra virgin olive oil

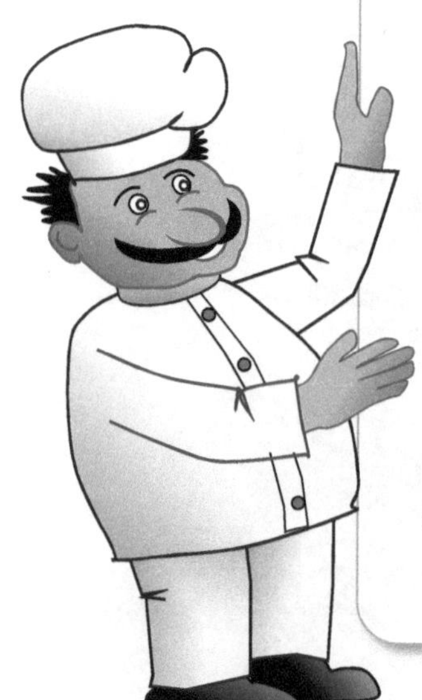

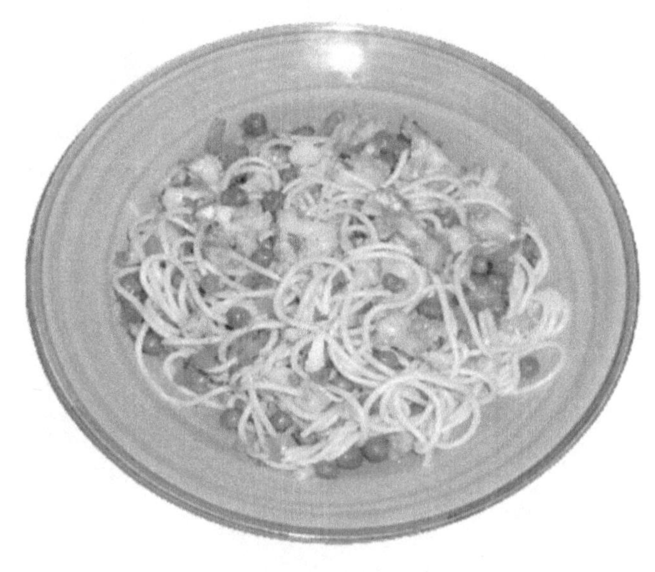

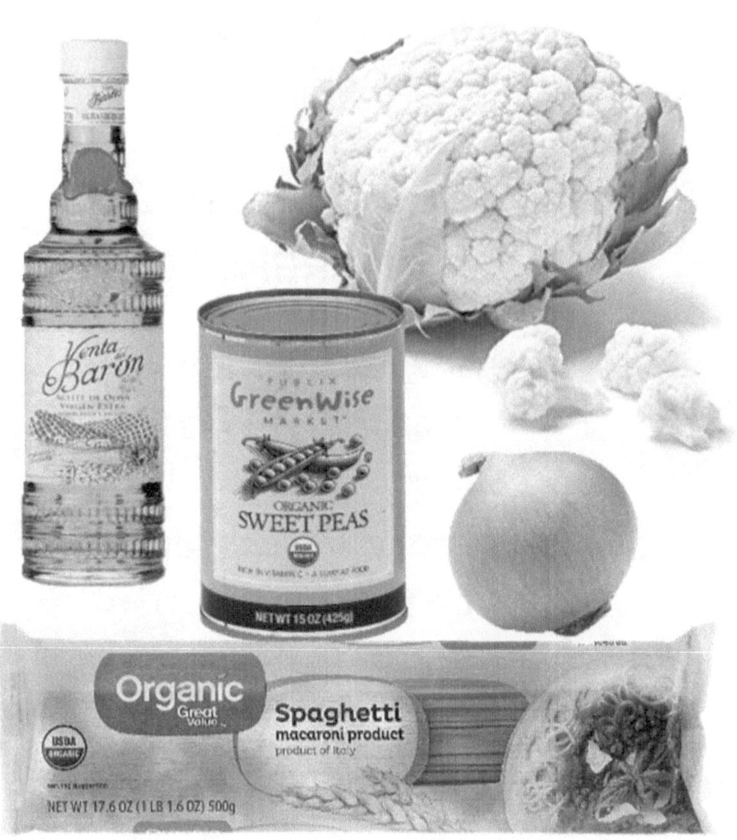
Venta del Barón
GreenWise
MARKET
ORGANIC
SWEET PEAS
NET WT 15 OZ (425g)
Organic
Great Value
Spaghetti
macaroni product
product of Italy
USDA
ORGANIC
NET WT 17.6 OZ (1 LB 1.6 OZ) 500g

PIZZA VEGAN SUPREME

1. Amy's Vegan
Supreme Pizza

(bake in toaster oven
or regular oven)

PIZZA VEGAN MARGHERITA

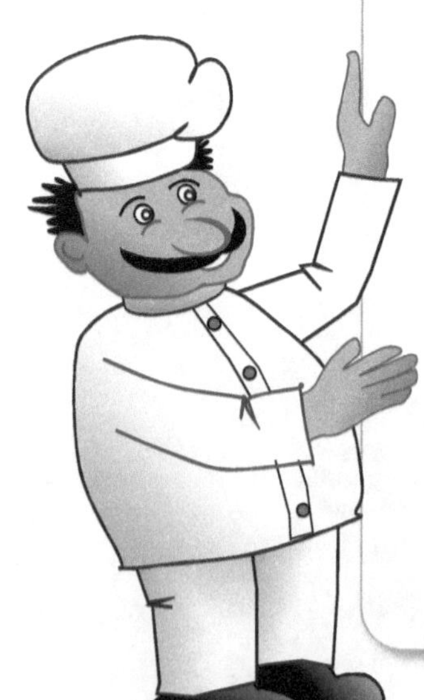

1. Amy's Vegan
Margherita Pizza

(bake in toaster oven
or regular oven)

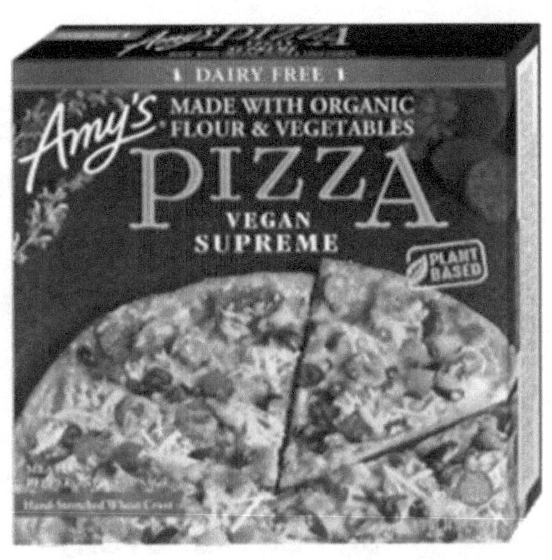
DAIRY FREE
Amy's
MADE WITH ORGANIC
FLOUR & VEGETABLES
PIZZA
VEGAN
SUPREME
PLANT
BASED

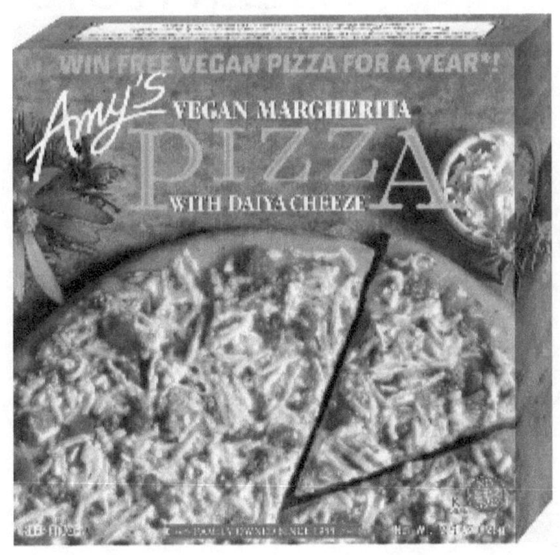
WIN FREE VEGAN PIZZA FOR A YEAR*!
Amy's
VEGAN MARGHERITA
PIZZA
WITH DAIYA CHEEZE

PIZZA ROASTED VEGETABLE (NO CHEESE)

1. Amy's Roasted Vegetable Pizza

(bake in toaster oven or regular oven)

PIZZA PESTO & ROASTED ARTICHOKE

1. Amy's Pesto & Roasted Artichoke Pizza

(bake in toaster oven or regular oven)

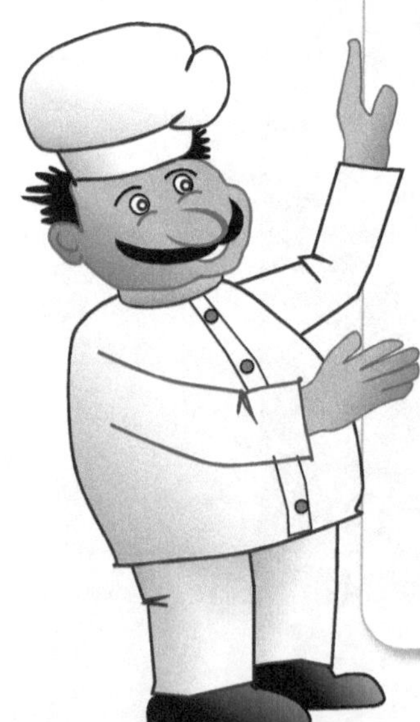

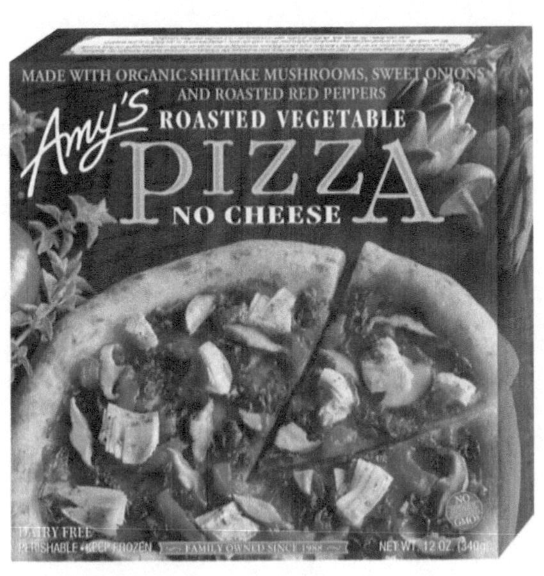

MADE WITH ORGANIC SHIITAKE MUSHROOMS, SWEET ONIONS
AND ROASTED RED PEPPERS
Amy's
ROASTED VEGETABLE
PIZZA
NO CHEESE
DAIRY FREE
PERISHABLE • KEEP FROZEN
FAMILY OWNED SINCE 1988
NET WT. 12 OZ. (340g)
NO
GMOs

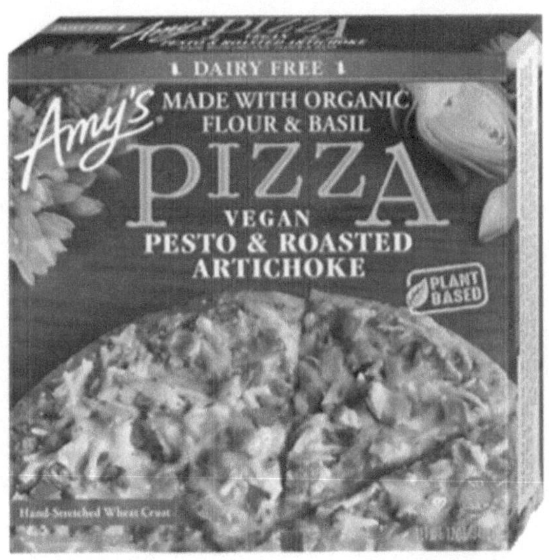

DAIRY FREE
Amy's
MADE WITH ORGANIC
FLOUR & BASIL
PIZZA
VEGAN
PESTO & ROASTED
ARTICHOKE
PLANT
BASED
Hand-Stretched Wheat Crust

HOLIDAY TURKEY DINNER

1. gardein Holiday Roast cranberry & wild rice stuffing *plus* gravy packs

2. organic Russet mashed potatoes

3. organic green beans

4. organic whole berry cranberry sauce

5. organic carrots

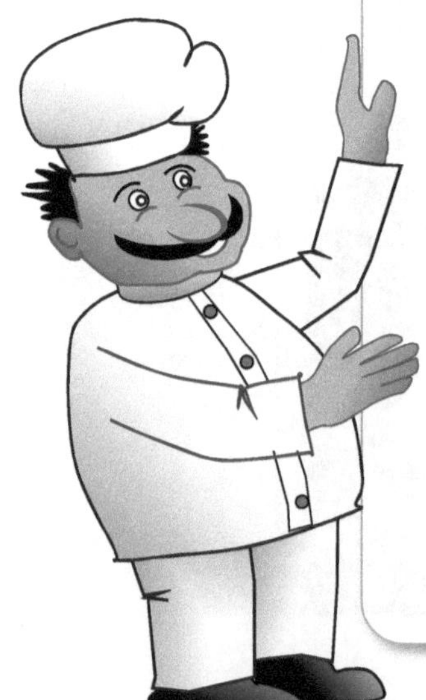

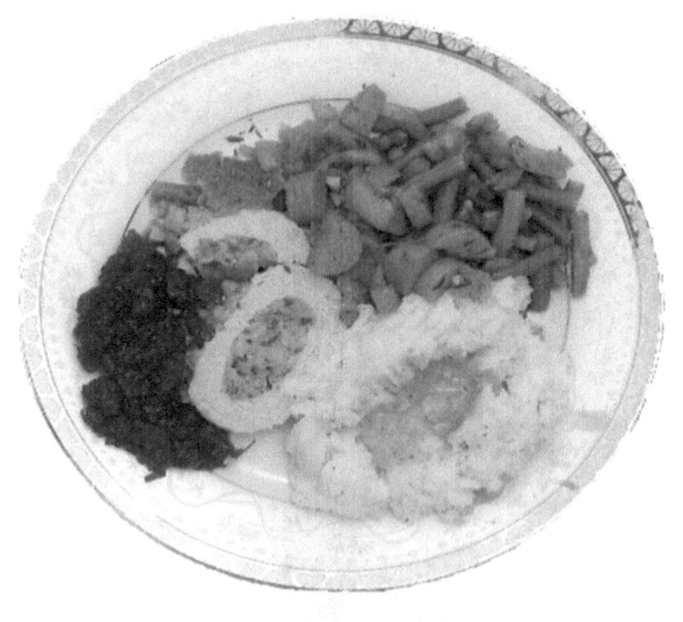

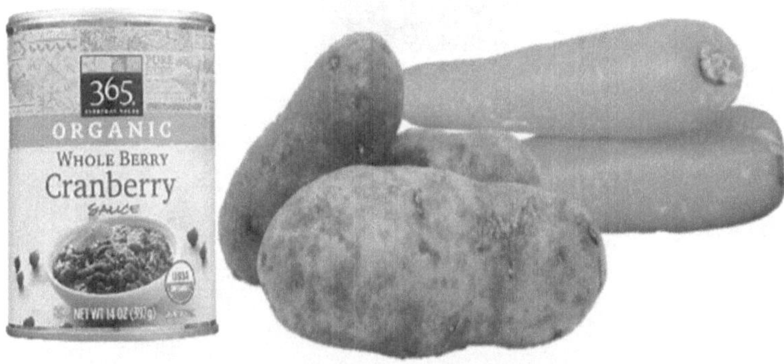

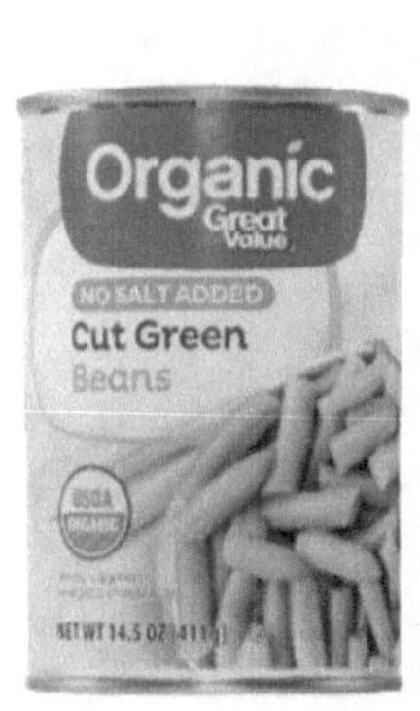
Organic
Great Value
NO SALT ADDED
Cut Green
Beans
NET WT 14.5 OZ (411g)

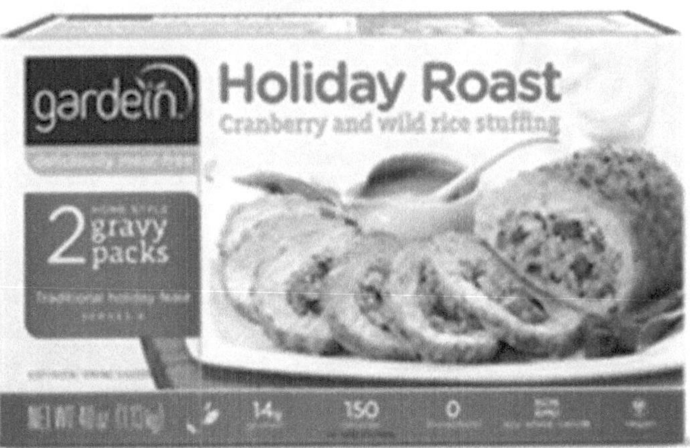
gardein
Holiday Roast
Cranberry and wild rice stuffing
2 gravy packs

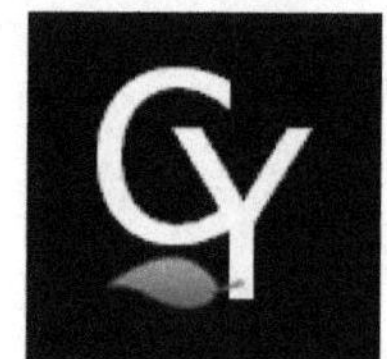